Dedica

Robert D. Terry

(1928-2004)

To alice,
Be healthy!

Alice
The Best to you
Health!

Alice
Good Luck with
our program
To your good Health

Contents

Modules

Introduction

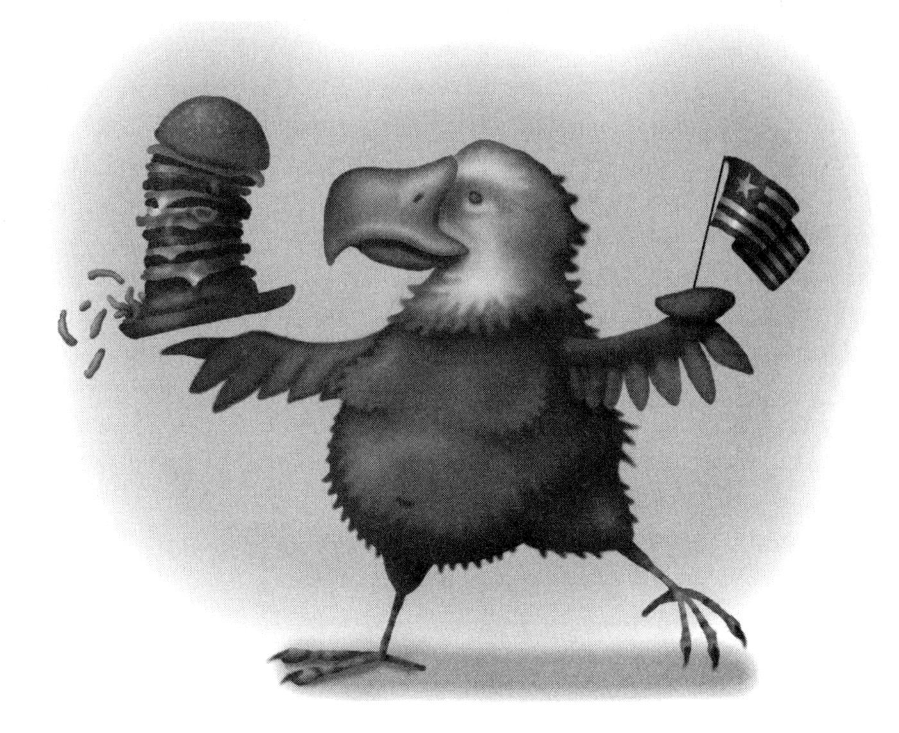

What this book IS NOT.

This is not a book about dieting. It's about starvation.

Starvation is a strange phenomenon to be playing a role in the 21st century in the wealthiest nation on the planet, but there is no other word for the culture of weight-consciousness and weight loss that pervades every corner of our daily life.

From skeletal models defining our concepts of beauty in the sensory overload of magazines, movies, and media, to the fat-free, zero-calorie choices on the supermarket shelves, to the rise in eating disorders among pre-pubescent girls and the increase of Type II Diabetes in the over-40 population, starvation is the silent culprit.

Self Help doesn't.

We have dozens of diet books on the self-help shelves of every bookstore, a weight-loss industry grossing 50 billion dollars in revenue every year, with 45% of the female population and 25% of the male population on diets at any given moment. Yet, according to the latest figures, 66% of American adults are overweight/ obese and 15% of our children are seriously overweight. This is costing a fortune in obesity-related health care and broken, despairing lives. And it's getting worse, not better.

This is not a coincidence. There is no logical way that using words like "sinful" to talk about eating certain foods, idolizing ultra-thin images, and applauding fat-to-thin celebrity stories the way our grandparents glorified rags-to-riches tales could not be related to the fact that we are growing increasingly obese. We are getting fatter, not despite the fact that we are encouraged to eat less, but because of it.

Americans are literally starving themselves into obesity, dieting more, and weighing more. We have truly become a "starvation nation."

What this book IS.

So, if this is not a self-help diet book, what is it?
To start with, it's a concise, readable look at the shocking news that our very attitudes, our social mores, our popular culture, and even misdirected aspects of our increasing attention to health are sabotaging our hopes and dreams of living fit, energetic lifestyles, as well as forcing whole segments of our population into at-risk eating behaviors and setting up a situation where even the best-intentioned dieters are doomed to failure.

Take Home Point:

- Dieting makes you fat.
- You can lose weight by eating.
- There are no such things as "bad" or "good" foods.

Chapter 1: YOUR Problem ... and How To Solve It

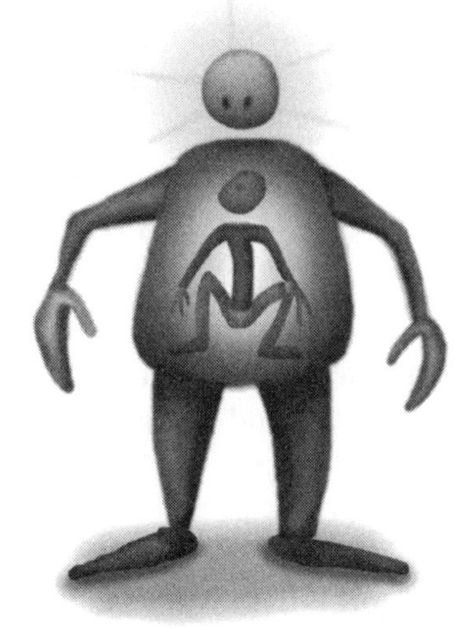

Let's get one thing clear. In your deepest heart, you must want to lose weight for good. You must want to be happier. You must want to live longer and healthier.

You must *want* to enjoy your meals and snacks MORE and not less. You must *want* the sense of confidence, pride and well being that comes with regular aerobics and exercise. You must admit the possibility that fad dieting is not going to work, ever, and learn the rock-solid reasons why that is so, as shown in this book.

The first step in any self-improvement program is to accept yourself and accept your bone structure, your body type, namely your genetic makeup, and your personality as it really is without any self-hating hang-ups about how you appear to others or in the mirror, or how much you weigh. These are things-- body type, bone structure, genes, your personality – that you cannot change. But tell yourself you're going to work on the things that you can change, which are your weight, if that's your problem, your personal health condition, your eating habits, your daily and weekly exercise, your excess poundage, and, finally and most importantly, the lifestyle that allows you to exist in the first place.

The second requirement is that you stop all fad dieting now--right now. Stop even thinking about dieting. Prepare to reject all future dieting magic bullets, drugs, "no this" and "no that" fad diets of any kind. There are no "new discoveries" on how to lose weight with or without dieting.

The third requirement is to start eating. Start eating well. Not tomorrow, not next week, but with your very next meal. Never starve yourself again. And you won't. Because this program will help you decide HOW to eat, HOW MUCH to eat, and WHEN to eat, but not WHAT to eat. You will make that choice. We will offer you alternatives to those suggestions. We will help you find your own alternatives, but we will never permit you to starve yourself again – and, when you see and feel the RESULTS to be gained by the following TOMORROW'S WEIGH® nutritional and exercise program, you will feel wonderful - about yourself, about your body, about your food, your sleep, your confident personality, and your exercise program. What's more, you'll be preparing, eating and enjoying all the food you need or want, for the rest of your healthy life!

Look at what is on the menu for your very next meal. Is it chock full of sugar? Is it something you know you can't stop eating, even though you are satisfied? Is it all highly processed? Is it a pickup from a fast food? Peek ahead to Chapter 3 and check your menu with what TOMORROW'S WEIGH® recommends you need to be eating. If possible, discard those destructive choices on today's menu. If not, enjoy your next meal whatever it consists of right now, because that's the way you will be enjoying your meals - even more so - after you get with the program. However, if it's processed, sugary, addictive or a fast food "quickie," let it be the last! Because you're going to change all that.

The fourth requirement is for you to be prepared to accept a regular exercise regimen. It might begin with just stretching, breathing, walking, swimming, and basic aerobics. Whatever it is, you should plan on having your physician's approval. Soon you will start the training necessary to discard excess fat and build lean muscle. Your heartbeat and your breathing will be quick to notice the difference and, most of all, you'll start to really enjoy it.

The fifth requirement is to get ready to limit your TV-watching, surfing the net, jumping in the car to go even a short distance, and relying totally on household gadgets for every single chore. As you well know, these things (except for the automobile) don't get you anywhere that you really want to go! If you have some limitations, you know how much you can do. Whatever your circumstances are, you can start to stretch, breathe right, pay attention to what you eat, enjoy it more and assume a style of living that leads to a longer and more fulfilling life. That is what this program is about, not only your "Tomorrow's Weigh®," but also your lifestyle today and tomorrow.

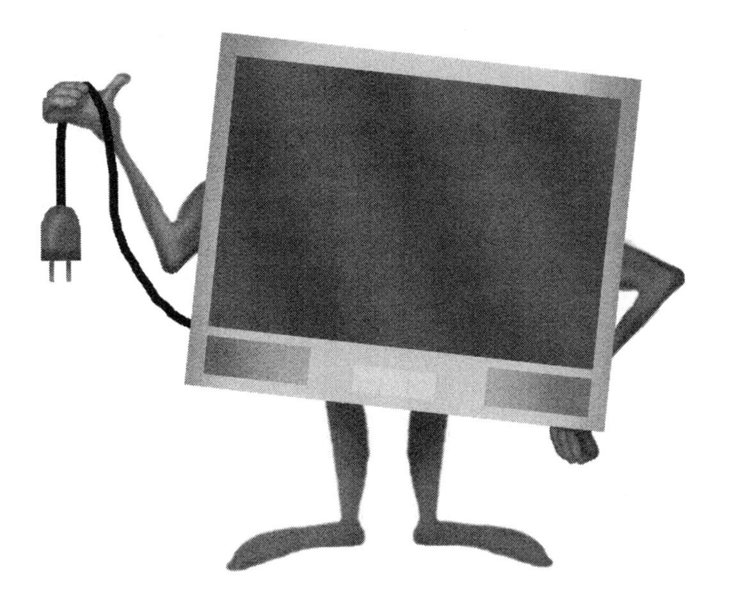

Take Home Point: Diets lead to short-term weight loss. To sustain weight loss, one must undergo a lifestyle change.

Why Diets Don't Work

When Dr. Ancel Keyes and his colleagues at the University of Minnesota began their study in the Fall of 1944, it wasn't dieting they were looking at. Keyes is the "K" in K-rations, and he was actually compiling data for the U.S. government to assist famine relief in Europe and Asia.

Keyes placed 32 conscientious objectors to the ongoing war--all healthy young men used to eating hearty meals--on a voluntary "semi-starvation" diet of 1570 calories a day. That's less than half of what they were used to eating but a lot higher than the 1000-1200 calorie fad diets touted today in most women's magazines!

The starvation program having ended at the six-month mark, their metabolism slowed with an average drop of about 40% at the end of six months. Additionally, they felt cold, weak, tired and became obsessed with food, even collecting recipes, planning menus and studying cookbooks! Further, they became depressed, anxious, irritable and anti-social toward others in the group. Within three months, they were eating normally again. They gained back more than half the weight they'd lost. They gained fat tissue instead of hard muscle and "soft roundness" began to be their body type. Yes, they had lost pounds, but it was coming back on as increased fat!

The men also became "binge" eaters. They could not seem to satisfy themselves and ate to the point of being stuffed. They not only gained their lost pounds back, but continued to overeat and gained additional weight well after the study.

As they continued to eat again, some of their symptoms went away. But long-term effects lingered, including binge-eating, disruption of their appetite at regulating center and other types of behaviors which would sabotage their weight balance well into the future.

Chapter 2: Why We Don't Recommend Fad Diets or Any Other Diet Plans

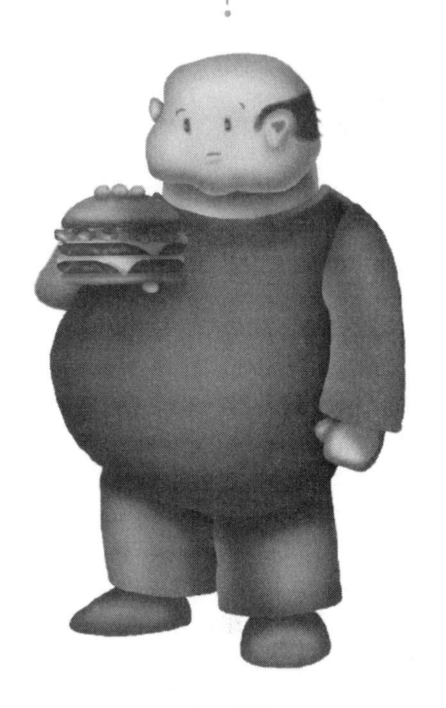

Diets are dangerous. In fact, some diets can be killers.

Any diet plan, other than a balanced wholesome one, either adds something which your body does not need, or, more often, deprives it of some of the things it does need. Food marketers, authors, columnists, and even doctors shout about "no fat," "low fat," "low carb," and "high protein" diets. However, take away those fats, those carbohydrates, and the proteins needed to nourish your body, and these "starvation diets" are life-threatening. They are life-threatening because either the body eventually dies of hunger, or it sustains irreparable damage from severe malnutrition, OR - after the diet becomes intolerable and regular eating resumes - they cause compulsive overeating. As a result, the body regains the pounds shed by dieting, plus more. Worse, the body usually stores both the restored and the new pounds almost entirely as fat, not as the lean muscle it may have lost in the diet phase!

Starvation diets take away what you need to renew your tissues, bones, muscles, skin and blood. They take away the energy you need to get through every day. Our bodies are designed to renew themselves, unless catastrophic illness, deprivation or WE OURSELVES interfere with that renewal.

Proteins, carbohydrates and fats are the essentials that every individual needs to stay healthy and grow their tissues, bones, muscles, skin and blood.

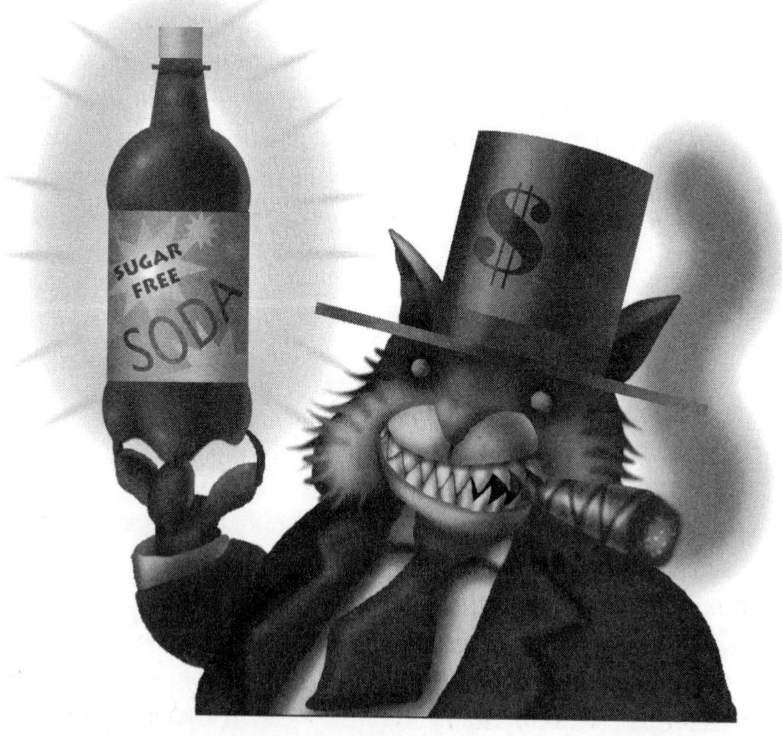

Meanwhile, huge food conglomerates with savvy marketing experts are having a heyday. They know a good thing when they see it on a sales chart. How about soft drinks? They are colored carbonated water, with "sugar-free" meaning that they may have no energy benefits, having chemical additives instead. The whole spectrum of diet products over the past 30 years has doubled, tripled and now quadrupled in sales. Book publishers can't put more diet books out on the shelves fast enough! Television hosts assault us with more "guests" with magic weight-loss formulas, books, commercials touting diet drugs, shakes, nutrition bars, drinks and "before and after" testimonials.

Frankly, if diets work, why is what we call "over-overweight" (obesity) on the rise? Why is there an epidemic of Type II Diabetes in children, teens and adults? Simply, the widespread phenomenon of fad diet after fad diet and the repeated myth of benefits are bought into by the millions. Many if not most of the diets are a form of starvation. Whenever a living thing, i.e., your body, loses something, nature assures that either that living thing will die-- OR, sooner or later, the process leads back to making up for that loss- in our case, by overeating and weight gain.

The flab problem goes way beyond shame, guilt and exhaustion. It causes people to make wrong decisions, such as going on a diet that utterly cuts out the needed balanced supply of proteins, carbohydrates and fats. An example is skipping meals, rather than eating wholesomely three- to- five- times a day. Another is lolling around, flopping down in front of the TV or computer screen for hours, without any exercise day after day, or being plunked in the driver's seat, not even walking as far as the mailbox on the corner. All the time, people think that they're solving their weight problems through "cutting calories" by using pills and diets!

Yet, is turning a steering wheel exercise? Is opening a car door, stepping into the passenger seat, exercise? Is taking that elevator or escalator one or two flights a form of exercise? Hardly!

In other words, just about every hour, every day, wrong decisions about how to lose weight cause people to become chronically tired and to become candidates for lifelong disease; and it's all because their bodies are starving.

You need a certain amount of energy just to live, to think, eat, sleep and breathe. The body is not like a furnace or stove which, when the fire goes out, just goes cold. Nature wants the body to live and survive whatever the circumstances. That's the whole purpose of life, and why we're immune to deadly germs, why we heal, and even why we reproduce. So when the fuel isn't there, the body instinctively goes looking inside itself for the energy to survive. First, it seeks out the vital "blood sugar," produced in your liver, because blood sugar fuels the most important organs in your body and your brain; and it serves the central nervous system. The survival of the brain and nervous system are the first priority of any sentient being. They are huge energy consumers compared to other parts of the body, and so they use up the liver as a source first.

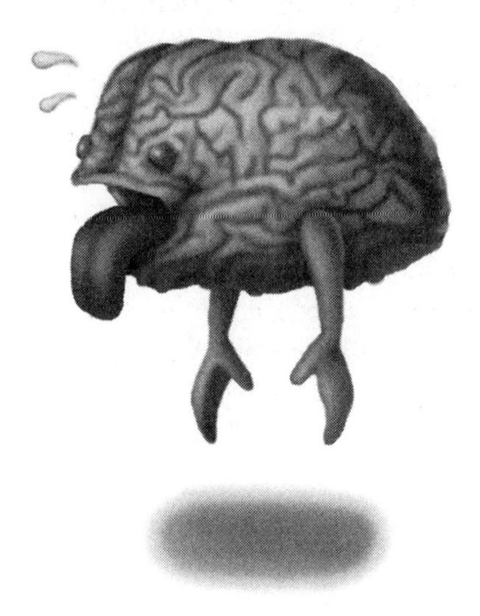

The brain has to go looking elsewhere to make more blood sugar. Where does it go? Not to the fat cells. They're good for energy for the rest of the body, but not for the blood sugar to use as "brain food." So, when the brain food isn't readily available from starches, dairy and fruit in a person's diet, and there's none remaining in the liver, then the brain goes looking for the tools it needs to make more blood sugar. Those tools are called "amino acids". Where does it find them? By breaking down the proteins found in the lean muscle tissues.

Before you know it, the body is in a state of what doctors call "ketosis" (see box below.) This is precisely what occurred to concentration camp victims in WWII. It seems horribly absurd, but that's exactly what some diet plans want to have occur to their victims today because it shows up as weight loss when the victim steps on the scale! After the bones, lean hard muscle is the heaviest part of the human body. For hucksters, less means more; it's money in the bank for them.

Ketosis is an unnatural state in the body. When the body is deprived of carbohydrates, the body looks to other sources, stored fats or triglycerides. These are broken down in the blood in the form of ketones. These ketone bodies tend to mask your appetite. Even though the brain may demand glucose, ketosis results. This may cause symptoms such as headaches, light-headedness and mental fatigue. Eventually, if you remain on a diet, it will deplete fat stores and breakdown protein from your muscles to maintain energy. The onset of ketosis is a semi-starvation state.

Take Home Point: Any diets that induce ketosis are unhealthy.

Chapter 3: What, When and How to Eat

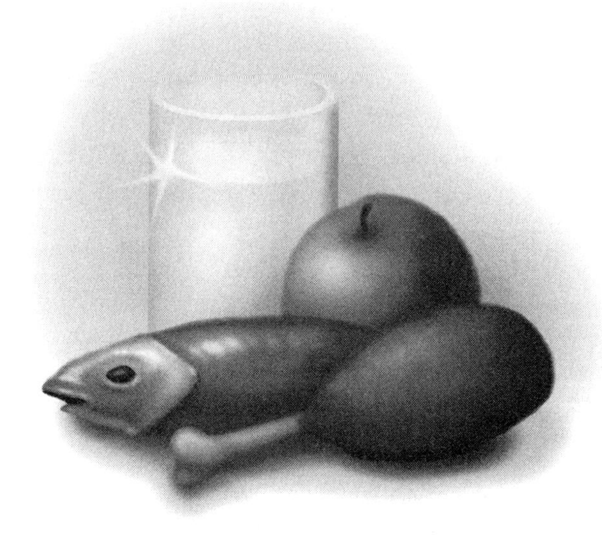

Nutritious eating is like standing up and not falling down; it's all about balance. Keeping your balance in nutrition is to strive for a balance of carbohydrates, proteins and fats. Yes, that's what we said first; carbohydrates: the very carbs which many diets try to take away from you!

Well, let's talk about that. Some dieters have lost a lot of

Low Carb High Protein Diets? Why not?

Much has been said and written lately about how the balance provided by carbs is unnecessary... that you need to restrict carbs, sadly to a dangerous level. Some dieters have come forward with spectacular short-term success stories, claiming the secret was this or that "high protein, low carb diet," but all these results were "short term." How about the l-o-n-g term? Isn't that what you're looking for?

weight on low carb-high protein diets, over the short-term, like six months. But nobody is offering any evidence of what the long-term effects of protein-heavy, low carb diets are! However, the nutritional experts do know. The fact is that the body can survive almost any nutritional program inflicted upon it, be it starvation, or obesity - but the one thing it can't tolerate forever is an all-protein diet. You don't need a nutritionist to tell you that sooner or later you need carbs to give you the energy to get all the things done which you need to get done, get the exercise you need, manage your weight and stay well! Carbs are so vital that they should make up at least 50% of your diet-- and come from the right sources.

Proteins are just as important as carbs. If you get enough carbs, you require about 20% of what you eat in muscle-building proteins. In fact, more is not good. Less is worse. Finally, fats are also important; approximately 30% of your calories should be in fats. Realize that fats are not the cause of the excess flab on your body. Just the opposite. Fats in a "keeping your balance" nutrition plan are needed to make the carbs and proteins go to the right places and help you remove the flab.

When it comes to eating different types of food, our bodies respond differently, depending on what we eat. You will probably find yourself with a sleepy feeling after eating carbohydrates. Proteins, however, make you feel more alert. That's why they're good to include at lunch and for a quick pick-me-up snack. Those peanut butter and jelly sandwiches we craved as kids turn out to be a good idea after all. Fats are what help make you feel satisfied or full, and that's why they need to be a part of meals as well.

TOMORROW'S WEIGH® gives you three sample nutrition meal planning charts: a 1,500-calorie chart, an 1,800-calorie chart and a 2,000-calorie chart. These charts are not meant to be followed but rather, to provide you a framework of what a meal plan looks like. For example, if you're young, active and not over-overweight, start with the 1,800-calorie plan, and, when you graduate to heavier exercise, go to the 2,000-calorie plan. If you're older and/or over-overweight, start with the 1,500 calorie plan, and graduate to the 1,800. The following charts tell you which foods provide the best sources of all three.

1500 CALORIE SAMPLE MENUS

MEAL	MONDAY	TUESDAY	WEDNESDAY	THURSDAY
BREAKFAST	3/4c. rice krispies 1 c. skim or 1% milk 1 slice whole wheat toast 1tsp. margarine 1 small banana black coffee or tea sugar substitute	1/2c. oatmeal 1c. skim or 1% milk 1/2 English muffin 1tsp. margarine 2tsp. light jam or jelly 2tbsp. raisins black coffee or tea sugar substitute	2 (4 inch) pancakes 1tsp. margarine 2tbsp. sugar-free syrup 8oz. nonfat yogurt 1/2c. applesauce black coffee or tea sugar substitute 1tbsp. liquid or 2tsp. powdered nondairy creamer	1/2 bagel 1/2tbsp. cream cheese 8oz. nonfat yogurt 3/4c. blueberries black coffee or tea sugar substitute 1tbsp. liquid or 2tsp. powdered nondairy creamer
AM SNACK	3/4c. pretzels 8oz. nonfat yogurt water	3/4oz. (2-5) whole wheat fat-free crackers 1oz. american cheese water	2 (4 inch) rice cakes 8oz. skim or 1% milk water	1/4c. dried fruit 8oz. skim or 1% milk; water
LUNCH	1/4c. cottage cheese 6 saltine crackers 1/2c. carrot sticks 1/2c. celery sticks 1/2c. cantaloupe 1/2c. honeydew 2tbsp. reduced fat salad dressing diet soda	1/4c. tuna with 1tbsp. reduced fat mayonnaise 1 slice rye bread 1 leaf lettuce 1 slice tomato 1c. salad with 1tbsp. low fat salad dressing 1 small orange crystal lite	1oz. light cheese 1 slice Italian bread 1tsp. margarine 1/2c. vegetable juice 3oz. (17) small grapes club soda	1/2c. cooked kidney beans 2/3c. brown rice 1/2c. cooked broccoli 1tsp. margarine 1 small apple unsweetened cocoa
PM SNACK	3c. microwave popcorn water	1/4c. dried fruit water	1 piece of fruit water	3 crackers 1tsp. peanut butter water
SUPPER	1 medium (3 oz.) pork chop 1/2 large baked potato 1 tbsp. sour cream 1/2c. cooked carrots 1tsp. margarine 1/2c. fruit cocktail water	1 small hamburger 1 hamburger bun catsup and/or mustard 1/2c. green beans 1tsp. margarine 1 1/4c. whole fresh strawberries water	1/2 whole chicken breast 1/3c. baked beans 1/2c. cooked corn 1tsp. margarine 1c. salad with 1tbsp. low fat salad dressing 3/4c. mandarin oranges water	1 unbreaded fish fillet 1/2c. mashed potatoes 1/2c. sweet potato 1tsp. margarine 1/2c. cooked brussel sprouts 1 fruit juice bar (100% juice) water

1500 CALORIE SAMPLE MENUS

MEAL	FRIDAY	SATURDAY	SUNDAY	
BREAKFAST	3/4c. cherries 1 slice rye bread 1tsp. margarine 1/2 large grapefruit 1c. skim or 1% milk black coffee or tea sugar substitute	1c. shredded wheat 1c. skim or 1% milk 1c. reduced calorie cranberry juice cocktail black coffee or tea sugar substitute	1/2c. cream of wheat 1 (4 inch) waffle 1tsp. margarine 1tbsp. sugar-free syrup 1c. skim or 1% milk 1/2c. pineapple juice black coffee or tea sugar substitute	
AM SNACK	3 graham cracker squares 8oz. nonfat yogurt water	3 ginger snaps 8oz. nonfat yogurt water	8 animal crackers 8oz. nonfat yogurt water	
LUNCH	4oz. tofu 1/2c. mixed vegetable (without corn, peas or pasta) 1 tbsp. soy sauce 4 (2/3 oz.) breadsticks 12 fresh cherries 1 tsp. margarine tonic water	1c. bean soup 1c. spinach greens with 1 tbsp. regular salad dressing 2 small plums sugar-free drink mix 1/2c. sugar-free gelatin	1 hotdog with bun catsup and/or mustard 1/2c. cooked sauerkraut 1 medium fresh pear diet soda	
PM SNACK	(1) 1 1/3oz. breakfast, sport or energy bar water	1c. vegetables 2oz. low fat dressing water	3/4oz. (9-13) tortilla chips 1/4c. salsa water	
SUPPER	1 grilled chicken sandwich 1c. salad with lettuce, tomato and cucumber 1tbsp. regular dressing 1/2c. peaches water	3oz. turkey 1/3c. bread stuffing 1/2c. mashed potato 1tsp. margarine 1/2c. wax beans 1/2c. pineapple water	3 oz. unbreaded veal cutlet 2/3c. brown rice 1tsp. margarine 1/2c. cooked beets 1/2c. raspberries water	

1800 CALORIE SAMPLE MENUS

MEAL	MONDAY	TUESDAY	WEDNESDAY	THURSDAY
BREAKFAST	3/4c. cornflakes 1 slice pumpernickel bread 1c. skim or1% milk 1tsp. margarine 1 1/4c. whole straw-berries black coffee or tea sugar substitute	1/2c. cream of rice 1/2 English muffin 1c. skim or 1% milk 1tsp. margarine 2 tsp. light jam/jelly 1/2c. orange juice black coffee or tea sugar substitute	(1)2 1/2" biscuit 1tbsp. honey 1/2 grapefruit (large) 1c. skim or 1% milk 1tsp. margarine black coffee or tea sugar substitute	1/2 bagel 1tbsp. regular cream cheese 1 small banana 1c. skim or 1% milk black coffee or tea sugar substitute
AM SNACK	2 rice cakes 8oz. nonfat yogart water	6 whole wheat crackers 1 1/2oz. cheese (3g. fat or less) water	3 ginger snaps 1c. skim or 1% milk water	3c. low-fat microwave popcorn w/2tbsp. grated Parmesan cheese; water
LUNCH	1c. tuna noodle casserole 1c. salad w/ lettuce, tomato, cucumber 2tbsp. reduced fat salad dressing 1 small apple	1c. (8oz.) lasagna 1c. cooked zucchini 1tsp. margarine 4 whole fresh apricots diet soda 1c. sugar free gelatin	1c. spaghetti w/ meatballs 1c. green beans 1tsp. margarine 12 sweet fresh cherries tonic water	1c. chili with beans 2c. salad with broccoli, cauliflower and mushroom 2tbsp. reduced fat salad dressing 1/2c. fruit cocktail crystal lite
PM SNACK	1c. reduced calorie cranberry juice cocktail 3 graham cracker squares water	1 fruit juice bar (100% juice) 8 animal crackers water	3/4oz. pretzels 1 medium fresh peach water	1-1oz. String Cheese 1 small orange water
SUPPER	1 chicken breast and wing, breaded and fried 1/2c. mashed potatoes 1tsp. margarine 1/2c. carrots 3/4c. blackberries water	4oz. salmon 2/3c. white rice 1tsp. olive oil 1tsp. margarine 1/2 cooked spinach 1 c. cubed cantaloupe water	4oz. ham 2/3c. baked beans 1/2c. brussel sprouts 1tsp. margarine 1/2c. canned pears water	4oz. roast beef 1/2c. boiled potatoes 1 slice Italian bread 1tsp. margarine 1/2c. asparagus 1c. raspberries water

1800 CALORIE SAMPLE MENUS				
MEAL	FRIDAY	SATURDAY	SUNDAY	
BREAKFAST	2 (4 inch) pancakes 1tsp. margarine 2tbsp. sugar-free syrup 3/4c. blueberries 8 oz. nonfat yogurt black coffee or tea sugar substitute 1tbsp. nondairy creamer	2(4 inch) reduced fat waffles 1tsp. margarine 2tbsp. sugar-free syrup 1 small nectarine 1c. skim or 1% milk black coffee or tea sugar substitute	1/2c. bran cereal 1 slice rye toast 1 tsp. margarine 1c. skim or 1% milk 2tbsp. raisins black coffee or tea sugar substitute	
AM SNACK	3/4oz. baked tortilla chips 1/4c. salsa 1c. skim or 1% milk water	1/4c. granola 8 oz. nonfat yogurt water	8oz. Lowfat yogurt water	
LUNCH	1c. macaroni and cheese 1c. tomato/vegetable juice 2 small tangerines unsweetened cocoa	1/4 of 12 inch cheese pizza thin crust 2 c. spinach salad w/ mushrooms 2 tbsp. reduced fat salad dressing 1 1/4c. watermelon diet soda	1/2c. tuna 2 slices whole wheat bread 1tbsp. reduced fat mayonnaise 1c. carrot sticks 1c. celery sticks 17 small grapes tonic water	
PM SNACK	1c. vegetables 2tbsp low fat dressing water	1/2c. frozen yogurt 1/2c. strawberries (sliced) water	1/3c. Trailmix water	
SUPPER	4oz. roast turkey 1/2c. mashed sweet potatoes 1/3c. bread stuffing 1tsp. margarine 1/2beets 1/2c. applesauce water	4 oz. lamp chop 1/3c. brown rice 1/2c. cooked broccoli 1 slice whole wheat bread 1tsp. margarine 1/2c. canned peaches water	4 oz. veal chop 1/2 large baked potato 1 tbsp. reduced fat sour cream 1/2c. mixed vegetables (without corn, peas or pasta) 2 small plums 1tsp. margarine water	

2000 CALORIE SAMPLE MENUS

MEAL	MONDAY	TUESDAY	WEDNESDAY	THURSDAY
BREAKFAST	1/2 bagel 1tbsp. regular cream cheese 1 small apple 8oz. nonfat yogurt black coffee or tea sugar substitute 1tbsp. liquid or 2tsp. powdered nondairy creamer 1/2c. orange juice	2 slices reduced calorie bread 1tsp. margarine 2 tsp. sugar-free jam or jelly 1/2c. apple cider 1/2c. bran cereal 8oz. skim or 1% milk 1/2c. canned apricots black coffee or tea sugar substitute	1 English muffin 1tsp. margarine 1 small banana 8oz. nonfat yogurt 1c. reduced calorie cranberry juice cocktail black coffee or tea sugar substitute 1tbsp. liquid or 2tsp. powdered nondairy creamer	1 slice whole wheat toast 1/2c. cream of rice 1tsp. margarine 1c. skim or 1% milk 1tbsp. raisins 1/2c. pineapple juice black coffee or tea sugar substitute
AM SNACK	8 animal crackers 8oz. skim or 1% milk water	3 (2 1/2 inch square) graham crackers 8 oz. nonfat yogurt water	3/4oz. pretzels 1c. skim or 1% milk water	2 (4 inch) rice cakes 8oz. nonfat yogurt water
LUNCH	1/4 of 12 inch (6 oz.) cheese pizza, thin crust 1 c. salad with lettuce, tomato, cucumber 1 tbsp. regular salad dressing 1 c. cantaloupe diet soda	2c. chow mein over 1/3c. rice or pasta 1/2c. cooked zucchini 1tsp. margarine 12 fresh cherries crystal lite 1/2c. diet gelatin	1/2c. tuna salad 1 slice whole wheat bread 1c. carrot sticks 1c. celery sticks 3oz. (17) small grapes 1tbsp. low fat salad dressing tonic water	1/2c. chicken salad 1 slice Italian bread 1c. salad with lettuce, cauliflower and broccoli 2tbsp. fat free Italian dressing 1c. honeydew club soda
PM SNACK	24 oyster crackers 1c. cream soup water	3 c. microwave popcorn with 2tbsp. grated Parmesan water	1/4c. granola 8 oz. nonfat yogurt water	1 (2 1/2 inch across) biscuit 1c. skim or 1% milk water
SUPPER	4 oz. chicken 1/3c. baked beans 1 large corn on cob 1tsp. margarine 1 c. homemade coleslaw made with reduced fat mayonnaise 1 1/4c. watermelon water	4oz. turkey 2/3c. bread stuffing 1/3c. mashed potatoes 2 tsp. margarine 1c. cooked carrots 1/2c. fruit cocktail water	4oz. sirloin steak 1/2 large baked potato 1tbsp. reduced fat sour cream 1 slice rye bread 2tsp. margarine 1c. cooked asparagus 3/4c. mandarin oranges; water	4oz. pork tenderloin 1c. sweet potato 1c. peas and pearl onions 2tsp. margarine 1 small nectarine 1/2c. diet gelatin water

2000 CALORIE SAMPLE MENUS				
MEAL	FRIDAY	SATURDAY	SUNDAY	
BREAKFAST	2 (4 inch across) pancakes 1tsp. margarine 2 tbsp. sugar-free syrup 1/2 large grapefruit 1/2c. grapefruit juice 8oz. nonfat yogurt black coffee or tea sugar substitute 1tbsp. liquid or 2tsp. powdered nondairy creamer 1tbsp. nondairy creamer	1 slice unfrosted raisin bread 1tsp. margarine 1/2c. frosted flakes 1c. skim or 1% milk 1 1/4c. whole strawberries 1/3c. grape juice black coffee or tea sugar substitute	2 (4 inch square) reduced fat waffles 1tsp. margarine 2tbsp. sugar-free syrup 2/3c. fruit juice blends (100% juice) 8oz. nonfat yogurt black coffee or tea sugar substitute 1tbsp. liquid or 2tsp. powdered nondairy creamer	
AM SNACK	1 (6 inch flour) tortilla 1oz. melted cheddar cheese water	1/4c. granola 8oz. nonfat yogurt water	3 ginger snaps 1c. skim or 1% milk water	
LUNCH	1 small chicken leg 1c. boiled potatoes 1/2c. cooked green beans 1tsp. margarine 1/2c. apple sauce unsweetened cocoa	2oz. American cheese 2 slices Italian bread 1tsp. margarine 1/2c. tomato or vegetable juice 1 kiwi diet soda	1/2c. cottage cheese 1/2c. pineapple 1c. raw red - green pepper strips 1tbsp. regular salad dressing sugar-free drink mix	
PM SNACK	1oz. pretzels 1c. skim or 1% milk water	6 saltine-type crackers 1/2tbsp. peanut butter 1c. skim or 1% milk water	5 vanilla wafers 1c. skim or 1% milk water	
SUPPER	4oz. broiled haddock with lemon juice 1c. brown rice 1c. cooked mixed vegetables (without corn, peas or pasta) 2tsp. margarine 1 medium fresh peach water	4oz. shrimp 1c. white rice 1tbsp. soy sauce 1c. cooked broccoli 2tsp. margarine 1/2c. canned pears water	4oz. meat loaf 1c. mashed potato 1 slice whole wheat bread 2tsp. margarine 1c. cooked spinach 1 fruit juice bar (100% juice) water	

Just as important as the balance is the timing, which means starting like you'd start anything else, at the beginning, with breakfast. Millions and millions employ the two lamest excuses in history: "I don't have time for breakfast" and "I'm not hungry."

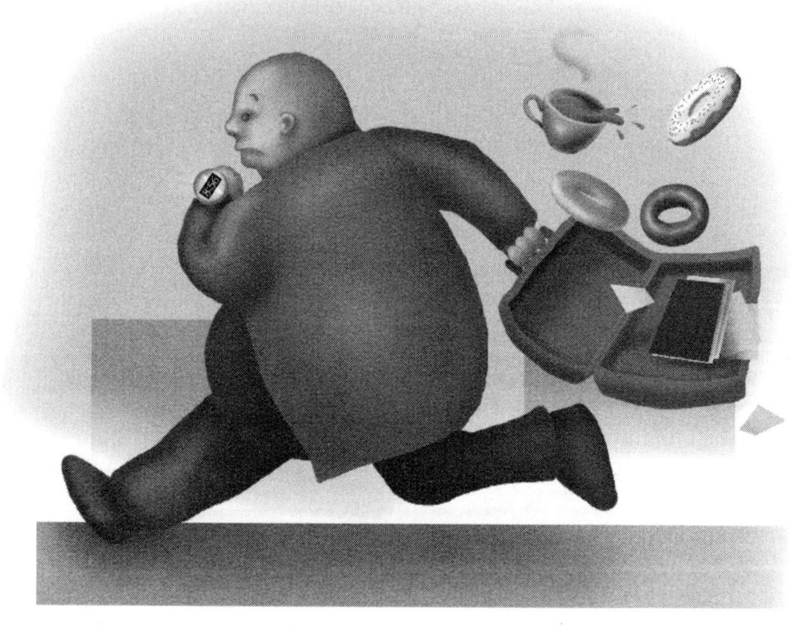

Of course they don't "have time" because they don't get up and do it. They may not be hungry because they stuffed themselves before bedtime to make up for the fact that they skipped breakfast yesterday and the day before that and that and that! And, by the way, don't fall for the nutrition bar scam, either. There are no substitutes for BREAKFAST.

Timing Means Taking the Time. One strong reason why you may not be "hungry"at breakfast time is because your tight schedule won't allow brief morning exercise, aerobics, jogging, or even a walk outside to work up an appetite. If you snatch a moment to "grab a bite" and then stuff it down, you are not taking the time to enjoy the daily meal you need most. By eating too fast, you may be uncomfortable all day. Take time to prepare something you like, chew thoroughly and enjoy every bite!

Typically these usually overweight, sometimes underweight, or even average-weight individuals gobble up a fast food "lunch". Ever watch a co-worker or a boss devour a hero sandwich and try to talk at the same time? It even makes you ill, not to mention that you have no idea what they're saying. Others do without the mid-day meal altogether, by surviving on coffee, soda drinks and sweets!

Many persons rush to run errands after the workday and gorge themselves at night.

That evening meal should be your lightest. Think of it as supper, not dinner. And make it relatively early. Remember the old adage that breakfast is like a king, lunch is like a prince, but supper is like a pauper. You don't need an abundance of calories to sleep, because you're not burning calories so fast.

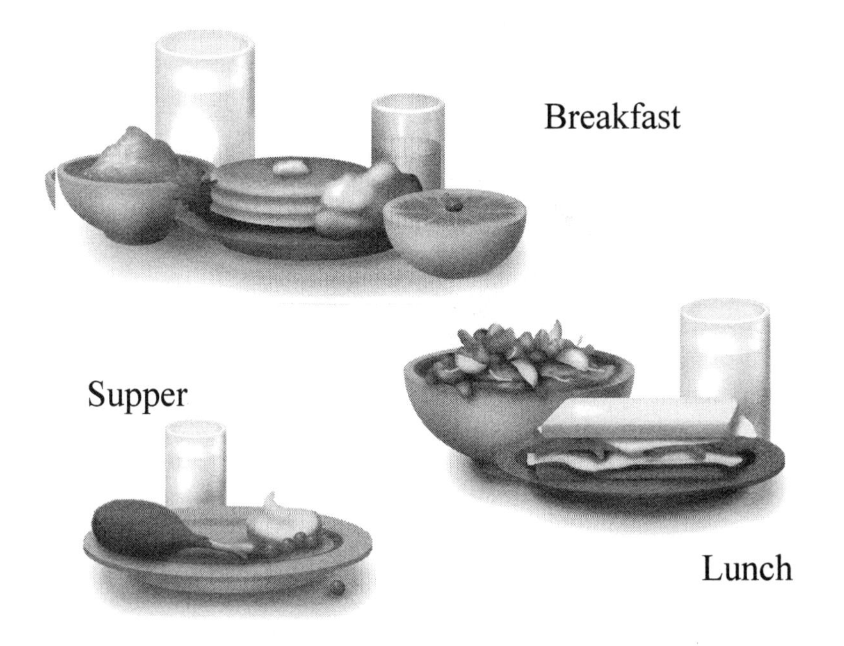

This is not to say you can't have a wholesome snack before you retire to bed, or a pick-me-up mid-morning or mid-afternoon for that matter. In fact, light snacks are a good idea, because you won't want to gorge at the nighttime meal.

Take Home Point:
If you want to lose weight, you must eat. You cannot lose weight or manage your weight successfully if you don't eat when your body signals that it's hungry. You need to pace your eating – not just meals, but snacks too - to coincide with your activity level at various points during your day.

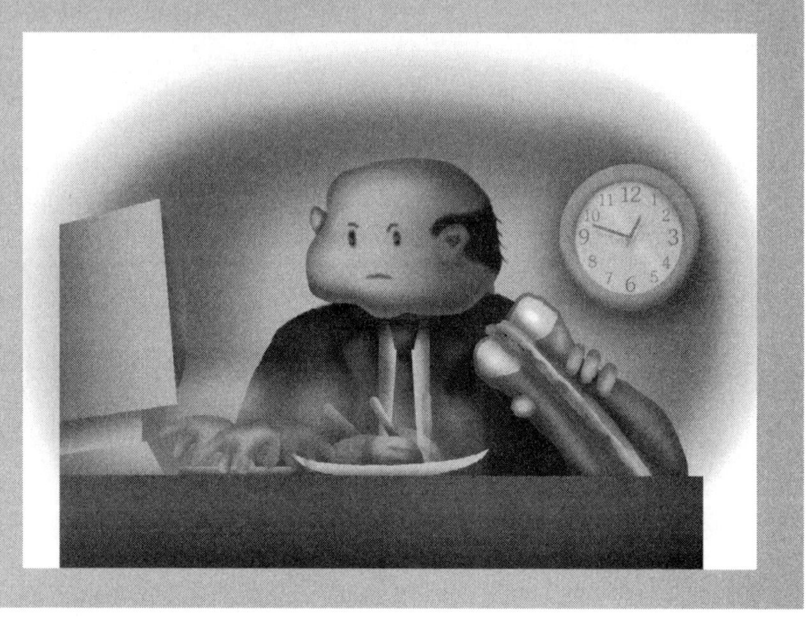

Chapter 4: The First Sure Way to Boost Your Metabolism

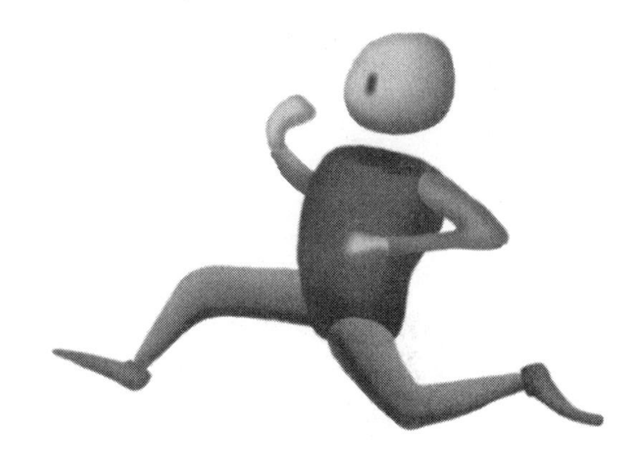

When a ship in days of old had too much ballast or cargo to weather a storm, the crew hollered, "Heave ho!" and disposed of the excess.

If a fully-fueled cargo jet loses an engine, and is so laden that it might go down, the crew jettisons everything that isn't of great value, and saves enough fuel to land safely.

Are you that ship or that cargo jet? Your mind, your vital organs and your lean muscles are of inestimable value. But your ballast or unwanted cargo isn't! If you can admit that without exercise you'll eventually sink or crash-land, you can "burn off" your ballast, your extra cargo, and not lose any of your essential organs, life-giving processes or muscle tissue.

Sometimes overweight people say, "Oh, my metabolism is just low." Some might truly have a low metabolism, but tests show that most of them don't. They just don't want to move, and moving happens to be the first key to everything else... Out of bed. Off the sofa. Out of the car seat! Away from the computer screen! Out of the lethargy!

You've seen the gimmicks and read the ads: Special supplements to help burn off excess fat. "My metabolism is too slow," goes the excuse for not being able to lose weight. "Metabolism" is the word we use for all chemical reactions that occur in our body, specifically how our bodies use food. And, yes, there is one sure way to spark your metabolism and get it to start burning fuel and producing energy. It's a three-letter word spelled: E-A-T!

Every time you eat, you set off chemical reactions that we call metabolism, the breakdown of food into substances that provide energy to every cell in the body. Not eating – or starving – slows the process. Eating speeds it up. Keeping your metabolism working properly does play a big role in whether you gain or lose weight.

Eating is something that is instinctive from the time we're born. It's a lot like keeping a fire burning. As the fire burns down, you have to keep feeding it to keep it going. Put on too much wood too soon, and you'll smother it. But if you wait too long or feed it too little fuel, the fire will just smolder.

Eating has to be an important part of the day, especially if you're trying to lose weight. Depriving the body of food or drastically restricting how much you eat will sabotage any weight loss plan in three important ways. First, it causes you to ignore your body's normal hunger cues and eventually leads to overeating. Second, it creates a feeling of being deprived, which your body and emotions naturally want to rebel against. And, third, it forces your metabolism to go into a starvation state, a kind of "Code Blue" where your body starts feeding on itself and slows the entire process down to preserve each precious calorie.

If you eat regular meals when your body tells you it's really hungry, you'll be eating at least once every four hours (or less time than that, if you get hungry sooner). And, after a while, you'll notice that your body begins to self regulate. Remember that 95% of all dieters fail to lose weight or keep it off. Dieting or starving is not the way to lose weight. Eating is.

WHAT IS YOUR BMI?

Instead of just looking at the traditional weight charts favored by insurance companies, nutritionists and other professionals have started to use another way of deciding when someone is overweight: the BMI, or body-mass index. This scientific ratio uses both height and weight to determine obesity. To determine your BMI, you divide your weight in kilograms by the square of your height in meters. One inch equals 2.54 centimeters and 100 centimeters equals one meter. One pound equals 0.45359237 kilograms. A BMI of below 20 is interpreted to mean that you have a low amount of body fat. The ideal, healthy amount of body fat will give you a BMI of between 20 and 22, while 22 to 25, although somewhat higher, is still considered healthy range. A BMI of between 25 and 29 puts you in the overweight range, while one over 29 would categorize you as dangerously obese.

But, like all charts that profess to determine the ideal, your BMI, while a good reference to have, is flawed. BMI fails to consider the lean body mass in its calculations, so that an athletic individual with low body fat and lots of lean muscle mass could be classified as obese using the BMI formula. Like all measurements, including weight, you need to consider your overall health and fitness to decide on the best eating and activity plan.

Take Home Point: If you don't eat, your metabolism slows down. This makes it harder for you to lose weight.

Chapter 5: Why and How to Increase the Rate at Which You Burn Energy

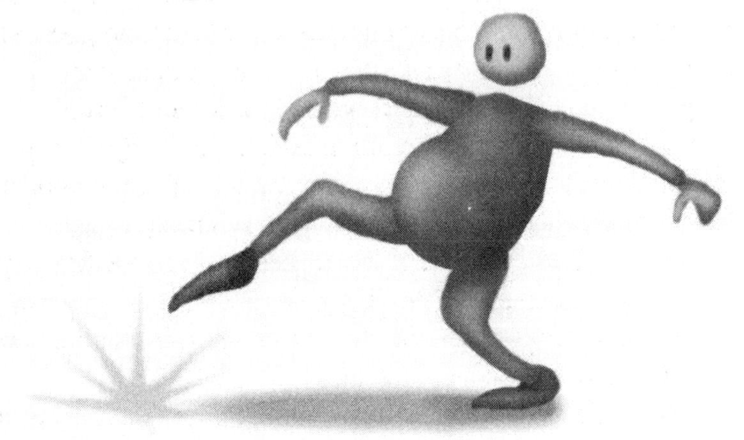

The longest journey begins with the first step. Walk where you'd otherwise drive or ride. Climb stairs where you'd rather escalate or elevate. When you escalate, you're escalating your weight over the long run. When you take an elevator, you're not elevating your metabolism! So, whenever you can, walk. Just take a scenic, neighborly walk, a minimum of 20 minutes a day.

Step two is to step into a bicycle seat, a real bike or a stationary one, and get the wheel(s) moving.

Step three is a dance step - or rather, many dance steps. Take lessons, or just call a partner and turn on the radio or CD! Do whatever moves you, because pretty soon you'll discover that moving is more fun than you ever thought.

Here are some other steps which you can take. Plant or tend a garden, or in addition to taking steps, take strokes-swimming strokes!

Those things are fun, but formal exercise is satisfying, and it makes you feel better, once you get into the habit. The purpose of formal exercise is to elevate the heart rate, i.e., to burn more energy.

How much formal exercise is enough? If you're starting, start light, with stretches and aerobics. Breathe in as you prepare to make the effort, and breathe out as you make the effort. You'll find yourself breathing deeper. You'll feel your heart beat faster.

You can do stretches and aerobics every day of the week-- but strive for a minimum of 30 minutes a day. As time goes on, some weight bearing is good, and, when you do start to include light weights, you still always start with stretches and aerobics.

Short of putting your health in serious jeopardy, however, there are really only two iron-clad ways to boost metabolism. The first, as we've outlined previously, is simply to eat. As long as you eat meals and snacks when your body needs fuel, you will keep the calorie burning process going. By satiating the appetite during those times of the day when you are most active, your body will store less energy as fat.

Even when you're being a couch potato or sleeping, your body is burning calories just to maintain your bodily functions and to keep you alive.

Metabolism is affected by three factors: eating, activity and resting. The amount of energy your body uses just to break down and digest your food accounts for 5-10% of your caloric need. Another 20-30% of the calories, or energy, you need goes to physical activity. But the most amazing statistic is the number of calories your body uses for its normal routine, such as breathing, keeping the heart pumping and all the other things your organs do. A full 60-70% of all calories consumed goes just to keeping you alive, which is known as your "resting metabolic rate."

A key thing to note about how many calories you need just to exist is that your body actually requires more calories to maintain muscle than it does fat. So, one second, surefire way you can "rev" up your metabolism and lose weight is by increasing your lean muscle mass. It's also the reason why it's sometimes easier for men to lose weight than for women; men naturally have more lean muscle mass than women.

As you age, your body gradually loses muscle and develops more fat, an unfortunate process biologists call "sarcopenia".

Studies show that muscle loss can begin as early as your 20s. In addition, if you've been dieting to lose weight, chances are that you've been losing not only fat, but lean muscle as well. If you've been on starvation diets – 1200 calories a day or lower - and/or high-protein, low-carbohydrate diets, most of your weight loss may be lean muscle. When you gain thc weight back that you've lost through dieting, it comes on as fat, reducing your lean muscle mass even more.

Muscle is the only part of your body which actively metabolizes fat. The more active your lean muscle is, the more calories you will burn throughout the day, whether you are running, sitting or even sleeping. So, obviously, if you want to lose weight, increasing your lean muscle mass and changing your body composition is the way to do it. Lean muscle is more dense and thus weighs more than fat, so the changes may not show up on the scale right away - which is another reason to stop obsessively weighing yourself. The good news is that muscle is about 22% smaller in size than fat, so what you can't tell by the scale, you can tell by the way that your clothes will fit as you develop more lean muscle.

Pound for pound, you will increase your metabolism and burn more calories by increasing your muscle-to-fat ratio. Nutrition experts have a rule of thumb for calculating the amount of calories needed to maintain and lose weight. Multiply your weight by 15. That equals the amount of calories your body needs each day to maintain its current weight – and it's probably a figure much higher than most people believe.

Now multiply your weight by ten, and that's the amount of calories you can consume and still lose weight. Both of these figures take into account the fact that your body is composed both of fat tissue, lean muscle and of course, fluids.

However, your body will burn more calories, even when you are at rest, if you build up your lean muscle. It takes about two calories per day to maintain one pound of fat tissue. But it takes between 25 to 50 calories to maintain a pound of muscle (Remember, your body by necessity is composed of both, so don't try using these figures to calculate your calorie needs!).

So, for example, if you put on 10 pounds of lean muscle while losing 10 pounds of fat, your weight would stay the same, but you will burn more calories every day, even while you're asleep!

Take Home Point: If you want to burn more calories and increase your metabolism, you should aim to increase your muscle mass. Pound for pound, muscle burns more calories than fat.

Chapter 6: Turning the Churn into the Burn

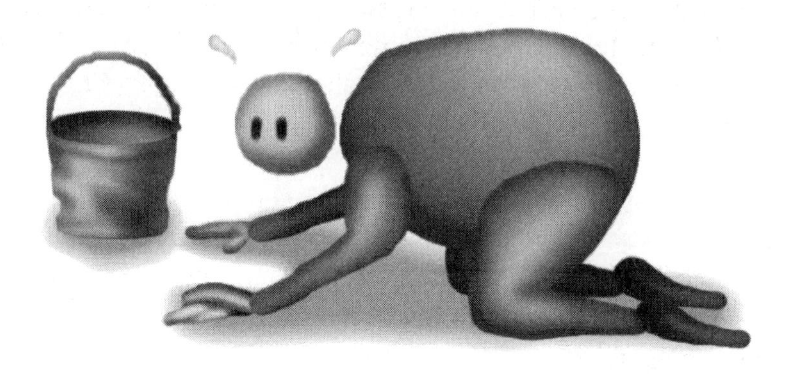

There are activities that we like to do which we can enjoy for exercise.

There's also another way to redefine physical activity. Even the experts are starting to take this into account in studies about fitness and disease. It includes, under the category of exercise, all those things which you do every day and adds them to the tally of how active you are and how many calories you've burned.

In this, our grandmothers and grandfathers had it all over us. Grandma would churn butter, do the laundry by hand and scrub the floor on her knees. Grandpa would chop wood, milk the cows and plow the field. Did they need to schedule a workout in order to get in shape? Ridiculous!

Yet, even in our computer age, there are still chores to do and routines which require physical exertion. The key, especially for the time-pressed, is to embrace these efforts as healthful movement and not as tedious work. The good news is that, once you start looking into how much exercise you can get from the kinds of activities you take for granted, integrating exercise into your day doesn't seem so impossible after all. Even though you didn't start out with weight loss, aerobic benefits and increased muscle strength as a goal, you get to enjoy all those advantages as well. So grab that hammer or dust mop and plunge right in.

Cleaning the house can burn between 200-300 calories an hour--more if you do it vigorously – as do feeding, dressing and taking care of your child, or repairing the plumbing. Ditto for raking leaves or sweeping the sidewalk or cleaning out the garage.

Like to dig in the dirt? Gardening can burn between 300-400 calories an hour. So can mowing the lawn (but not with a riding mower!). Raking leaves burns between 200 and 350 calories an hour. Shoveling snow uses 300-500. Dress warmly, in moisture-wicking layers, for any cold weather work or play. If you live or work on a farm, you have a big advantage. Planning a move? Carrying furniture and boxes of belongings back and forth to the truck, or up and down the stairs, can burn between 400-600 calories an hour.

You can increase the benefits of exercise by purposely making life a little tougher on yourself, too, such as parking at the far end of the mall and walking to the store. Eliminate competition for that parking space closest to the entrance of the mega-mart. Even choosing to shop the super stores can provide you with some benefits as you browse the spacious miles of aisles. You can also use the stairs instead of the escalator or elevator. And, just for a change, take the dog out before he whines and scratches at the door.

The calculations need not stop once the chores are done. When you consider exercise, you should begin including those fun, leisure pursuits which you may not normally think of as effort. A simple game of darts will use 150-200 calories an hour, while ping-pong or table tennis will burn between 200-300. Horse-back riding uses 200-300 calories an hour. How about badminton or playing golf? Both burn between 200-400, as does an hour of moderately-paced dancing. Ice-fishing in the winter, and stream fishing in the summer each burn 300-500 calories, while ice skating gives you a great benefit at 400-600 calories per hour. Even something as easy as bowling or a friendly game of Frisbee can burn nearly 200 calories an hour. The idea is to start moving and to keep moving as much as possible. Then watch the calories burn away.

Those who are overweight may feel at a disadvantage when it comes to exercise, but the truth is that, the more you weigh, the more benefit you'll get from exercise. The more you weigh, the more calories you'll burn doing the same activity as someone who weighs less. And the more intense the activity, the greater the benefit for those who weigh more. For example, take riding a stationary bike with a moderate amount of effort. If you weigh 130 lbs. you'll burn 413 calories an hour. At 155 lbs., you'll burn almost 500 calories, and if you weigh 190 lbs., and ride at the same pace, you'll burn a whopping 600 calories an hour--nearly 200 more calories than your slender counterpart!

For moderate walking, say 3 miles per hour, about how fast you'd go if you were walking your dog, a 130-pound person would burn 207 calories, at 155 pounds, you'd burn 246, and at 190 pounds, you'd burn 302 calories, 100 calories more per hour. If swimming is your exercise of choice, the numbers are even better. For moderate-to-light freestyle laps, you'd burn 472 calories an hour if you weighed 130-pounds, 563 if you weighed 155-pounds and 690 if you weighed 190-pounds.

It's one more reason why, no matter what you weigh or how overweight you might be, you can benefit tremendously from starting even a simple, moderate exercise program and keeping at it.

Take-Home Point: Obvious as it may seem, many people overlook the exercise benefits of routine chores and the pursuit of leisure. Anything that will get and keep you moving more can provide health benefits and even burn fat.

Chapter 7: Weights--Not Just for Male Bodybuilders

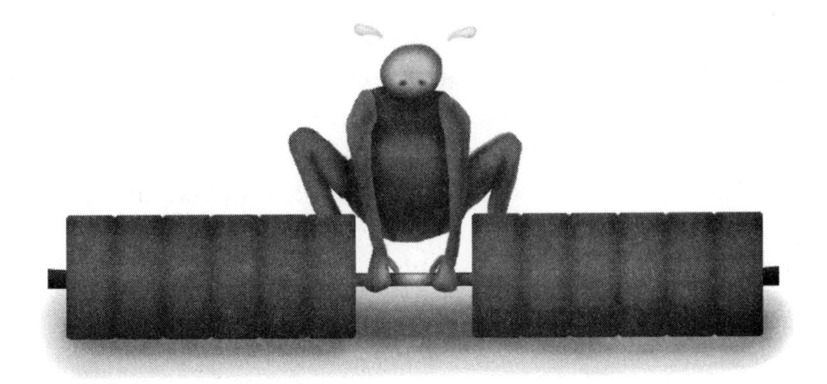

"I don't want to have those bulging muscles!"

That's still the usual reaction when you mention weight training to most women. But images of oiled down, vein-popping, flexing bodybuilders aside, adding weight training to an exercise routine is one of the best ways to see faster results and change your metabolism by changing your body composition from one of mostly fat to mostly muscle. The current term for it is strength-training, used interchangeably with weight training, and it is far and away the best addition to your overall fitness plan.

Strength training involves the use of resistance and weights, either with machines designed to work specific muscle groups efficiently or with free weights. Either type will produce results. Best of all, only a modest amount of strength training is needed to achieve big benefits. In addition to the calories you burn while training and the lean muscle you build which increases your metabolism, working with weights can produce "afterburn" -- increasing your metabolism for up to 15 hours after your workout. Aerobic exercise, while essential for cardiovascular health, doesn't keep the burn going as long. The main reason why building lean muscle burns more calories at a higher rate over a longer time is that, during weight training, you are actually tearing down muscle. Then later, when you're at rest, your body has to repair the muscle by building it up. This uses up more calories, which your body takes from your fat stores. This newly formed muscle tissue also uses more calories, even at rest, so it's a win-win all around. Another benefit is that, as you build more muscle, your body also builds more bone mass to support it. That's especially welcome news to older women concerned about losing bone mass through osteoporosis. And all this is true even with modest amounts of strength training. This kind of workout can also be convenient for those with limited time to exercise. While the "30 minutes each day" rule for moderate activity holds true, your body reaps the best results from weight training if you work muscle groups every other day or every two days, giving your muscle resting time to repair itself in between.

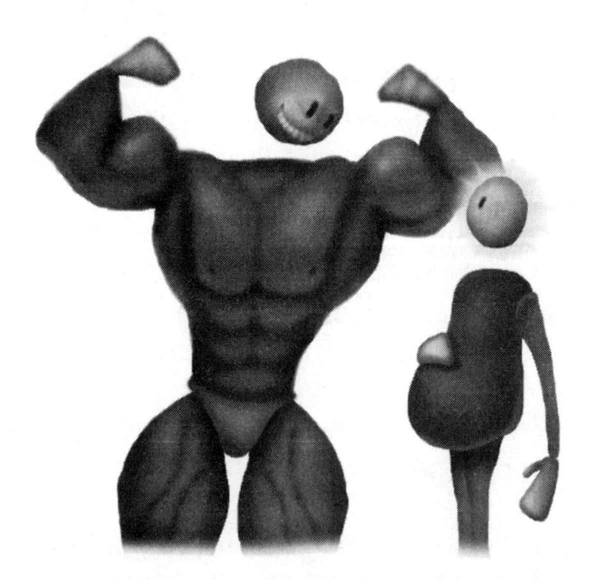

As for those fears of bulging, rippling muscles and popping-out veins, they are far-fetched. Most competitive bodybuilders who sport such physiques work out with mega-weights for many years to achieve such results. Some have also used steroids, which are harmful, health-wise. Nearly any body type can benefit from increased muscle tone.

Building lean muscle replaces what your body naturally loses through the aging process (which begins in your 20s!) as well as any lean muscle you may have reduced during past weight-loss attempts. It burns fat and increases your metabolism even at rest. It increases strength and flexibility and is easy to add to your workout plan. Strength-training, not diet fads and weight loss pills, should be the real health and fitness secret making headlines today.

Ever since strength training started gaining ground for its fat-burning and fitness potential, studies have been reporting other health benefits among a variety of age and population groups. A study done at Tufts University looked at knee pain in those over the age of 55. Half of those studied engaged in a home-based strength training program involving a set of exercises three times a week, while the other half concentrated solely on nutrition training. Those who did the strength training reported a reduction in knee pain and also better physical functioning overall plus improvements in quality of life and self-sufficiency.

Another study, this one of men over the age of 75, was even more striking. The subjects started a strength training program because their muscles were weak. They did eight-repetition power lifts only twice a week, adding more weight as they got stronger. At the end of one year, their performance had improved at least five-fold. Some of the men were lifting 600 pounds! Those who walked with the use of canes before beginning the program no longer needed them. Without question, strength-training needs to be included in senior health programs along with exercise routines for any age group.

Take-Home Point: Building lean muscle mass through simple weight training is the best overall way to boost your metabolism and manage your weight. But remember, you need both aerobic activities such as walking and jogging along with strength training to be successful in keeping fit and burning fat.

Chapter 8: 25 Excuses Not To Exercise–and Bursting Them!

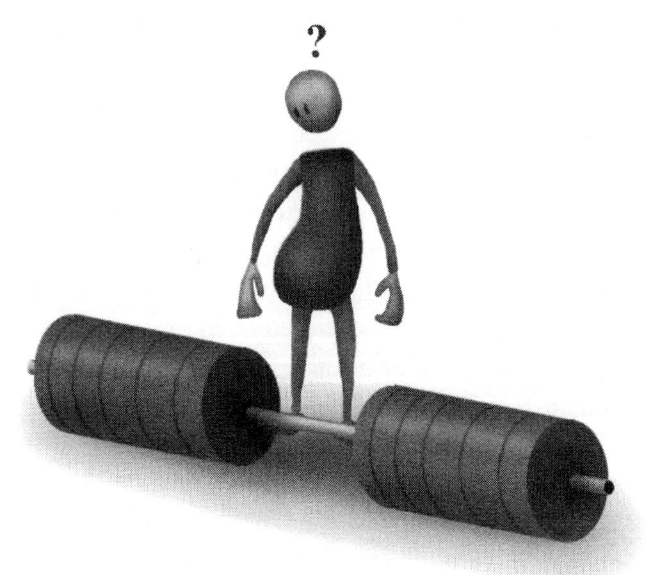

"A body at rest tends to stay at rest."

That basic axiom was used by many a science teacher to explain the principle of inertia, but it might just as well be the motto by which a majority of the population lives. The truth is that it's hard to give your body enough exercise after a tough day, even when you know you should and even when the desire is there.

There's no magic formula to exercising. Everybody knows they should, but it's just easier to come home, plop down on the couch and surf the remote. Or maybe you're a busy professional trying to juggle work and your life, or the demands of family. Spend an hour at the health club--who has the time or the money? Except for those who are fortunate enough to work at a profession that affords regular physical activity, the rest of us have to find some extra-curricular way to work exercise into our lives.

But you don't have to start by trying to run a marathon or bench press 500 lbs. In fact, trying to do too much too soon is the main reason why a lot of exercise programs fail over the long term. There are some simple ways of gradually working more activity into even the busiest of schedules, as well as some self-motivating techniques to defeat the exercise resistor that tends to dwell within us all.

The first step is to identify the particular forms of resistance within your own psyche. Inactivity is just a habit and, like many bad habits, our brain works hard to find ways to rationalize what we know isn't good for us.

Once you know your own inactivity excuses, the next step is to engage yourself in an all-out debate to break through such resistance and get that "body at rest" moving again. Here are 25 of the most common excuses and good arguments to counter them.

1. "I don't have the time." Nobody has the time to exercise--we have to carve out the time. Look for particular inactive times during the day and try to reduce them, or incorporate exercise into other activities. You could walk on a treadmill while watching TV, or lift three-pound weights while talking on the phone. Many fitness clubs have begun to offer 30-minute routines for busy professionals. Even a 15-minute walk could help you achieve your daily fitness goals. You could get up a half-hour earlier or take a short walk instead of a coffee-and-doughnut break.

2. "I'm too tired." Exercise can actually energize you and, over the long term, will increase your energy level. The trick is to find the time of day when your energy level is at its peak and use it. Eat enough to fuel your fitness routine.

3. "I hate the gym." Go for a walk, ride a bike, jump rope, rollerblade, go dancing, play catch, shoot some hoops, play volleyball, march around the house, rake leaves, clean the attic, get out on the golf course. There are so many ways, other than a gym or a health club, to get moving. Find something you like to do and have some fun.

4. "I'm not strong enough." Start slowly and work up to higher levels of activity. Even if you start with a short walk or by lifting

one or two pound dumbbells, sticking with it over a period of time will strengthen your muscles and allow you to work up to more strenuous exercise.

5. "I don't need to." Even if you're at your ideal weight, fitness is a concern for everyone. Especially as we age, maintaining a moderate level of activity is important to keep your muscles in working order. Recent studies show that even obese people can improve their health and decrease their risk of disease with regular exercise, while those at their ideal weights who don't exercise increase their risk of health problems.

6. "I'm not good at anything." It takes no special skill to walk, jog or run. Riding a bike is something most of us learned as children. And most health clubs and classes provide free instruction on their machines when you join--and, if they don't offer it immediately, you should demand it.

7. "I'm too old." You're never too old to exercise. A study of men in their 70s who began to do regular moderate weight training increased their strength by as much as two-thirds. And it's not unusual today to see 60, 70, 80 and even 90-year-olds swimming, walking, jogging and running marathons!

8. "It's too boring." Once again the secret is to find something you enjoy doing and to vary your routine when you hit the boredom plateaus. Been jogging every morning? Take the basketball and go shoot some hoops. Try hitting the fitness club during lunch or at a different time of day. If you use an indoor treadmill all the time, go for a walk outside instead. Buy books on tape and listen to a mystery novel or your favorite upbeat music while you work out. You can also make little games out of your routine or use interval training, which alternates short bursts of high intensity activity (i.e. two minutes of running) with longer stretches of lower intensity work (five minutes of walking).

9. "I'm hungry, I just ate, or, exercise makes me overeat." Have a small snack before working out to fuel the activity and if you feel full, wait until you feel more comfortable. You should also stay

hydrated, that hunger may actually be thirst. Over the long run, exercise actually helps keep your appetite in check and can be especially helpful in reducing those sugar cravings.

10. "My family needs me." Your family needs you healthy more! If all of your time is spent tending to the needs of others, you need to make a priority of your own needs more. Exercise can be your time to savor your solitude, and guarding your workout time is not only good for your body, but for your mental health as well.

11. "My job involves travel." Most hotels have some sort of fitness equipment on the premises for their guests. If the one you're staying at doesn't, many health clubs offer day passes at modest prices for travelers. Even airports are starting to recognize this need and provide fitness possibilities for flyers. You could also take a walk as a way of getting to know the area to which you're traveling; some cities have tourist walks complete with maps. Nearby shopping malls can also provide an aerobic walk and, in a pinch, going from one end of an airport terminal to the other end (without using the people mover) is usually enough of a walk in itself.

12. "I'm too stressed out." Exercise is the single most effective stress-buster known. Walking is especially good for dealing with stress; swimming can be relaxing and lifting weights or running are good ways to deal with anger and anxiety.

13. "I can't afford it." You don't need to become a VIP member of an exclusive club to create a fitness routine that works. Walking is free. Other ways to offset the costs of working out are to investigate public schools and park facilities, continuing ed. classes, church groups and the local Y. And don't forget garage sales and flea markets for bargains on used exercise equipment.

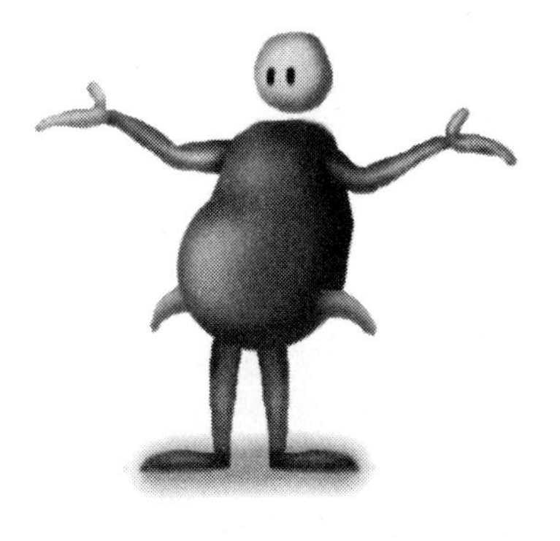

14. "I'm too embarrassed." It does take courage to begin a new activity and, if you're out of shape, it can be hard to be surrounded by hard bodies in spandex. But nowadays there are many more choices. You could hit the club at slower times of the day, or try something like mall-walking, where you'll blend in with the crowd. If you find yourself comparing your shape or abilities to others, don't. Think of all the people who are sitting around not making the effort and congratulate yourself for getting started. Have realistic goals and compete only with yourself. And remember, like any new habit, it gets easier as you keep doing it.

15. "I don't have the right clothing." Wear what you feel most comfortable and focus on the feel of the activity and the way you're improving each day. If it makes you feel better and gives you more motivation to buy an outfit just to exercise, pick one that fits your budget and flatters your figure. But don't let your wardrobe dictate your motivation.

16. "I don't have the right equipment." If you want to engage in complex rock climbing, it's important to have the correct equipment. But if your goal is to get moving, most forms of fitness require nothing more than your own body and determination to achieve results. Fitness centers and health clubs replace their equipment with the latest technology in order to attract new members, but you can improvise. Fill plastic bleach bottles with sand or water and you've got instant weights to lift. And bargains abound in garage sales, second-hand sports shops and large discount warehouse stores.

17. "I can't keep up with those instructors." You don't have to. Most fitness centers offer low-intensity classes as well as high intensity workouts. And even in a "one-workout-is-good-for-all" class, you can tone down the intensity of any movement to suit your level of fitness. Remember that you're competing with yourself only.

18. "I have to miss a day (or week, or month). " The demands of life can interfere with even the most carefully planned routine. You get a cold, have an urgent family matter or face an especially

hectic week. The trick is to get back to some sort of exercise routine as soon as possible. Don't let an inactive stretch become the excuse not to work out. Show up as if you never missed a day, but be careful to begin slowly or at a previous level and work back up over a period of time.

19. "It's too complicated." Walking is the simplest activity known to mankind and can be an extremely effective form of exercise. If you want to try something more complex, the best way is to take a class or two to see if you like it and learn the proper technique.

20. "I hate to exercise alone." Having an exercise partner is great motivation, but there are other ways to keep from being lonely. A class or a club, such as a mall-walking group or bike club, can put you in touch with new friends. Walking or running with a pet is also a good way to work out. But if all else fails and you find yourself going it solo, you can always use the time to savor your own solitude and work your mind along with your body.

21. "The weather is bad." Walkers can switch to indoor malls to keep the routine going or maybe you can vary your activity with the season, rollerblading in the fall, tennis in the spring, swimming in the summer, or a fitness class when the snow flies. You can also see the weather as a challenge to increase your determination. Did you ever feel a refreshing mist as you jogged or increase the intensity of your steps as you trudged through snow? Remember to dress for the climate and rely on layers as the weather gets colder and to keep well-hydrated, especially in hotter months.

22. "My body aches." You need to begin any exercise program slowly and gradually build up your strength and intensity over a period of time. Doing too much too soon will result in aches and pains, but beginner's soreness usually disappears as you keep working out consistently. For weight training you need to rest your body for two or even three days between working the same muscle groups. If you have a condition such as arthritis, swimming can provide the kind of exercise that is easy on the joints.

23. "I can start tomorrow." And the day after that or the day after that. Procrastination is just another bad habit that can be unlearned by going ahead and doing what you're trying to avoid. Tell yourself you'll work out for 15 minutes only. Keep your sneakers in your car or carry them with you. Make an appointment with yourself and write it on your calendar or daily organizer as if it were a meeting you could not miss. If all else fails, rely on Nike's slogan and "Just do it."

24. "I get winded just taking the stairs!" You will at first, but if you stick with some sort of regular fitness routine, you will improve over time. Don't try the 5 K run right off the bat. Walk around the block today, two blocks tomorrow, three the day after that. Try one flight of stairs and as you improve, then work up to two. It's a law of all exercise that the more you do, the more you can do and time is always on your side.

25. "Exercise never works for me." It's a familiar story. You're going along fine and then you get on the scale and you haven't lost a single pound. "Forget this," you say". Where's the TV remote?" It's important to put your motivation in perspective. Remind yourself that you're working out to become fit, not just to lose weight. Throw the scale away and go take a walk. Focus on how good it feels to move--you are doing an activity you enjoy, aren't you? It's nearly impossible to notice small improvements in your strength, fitness level or day-to-day ability, so record your progress in a notebook, but don't obsess over it. Look back after six months and celebrate how far you've come. Reward yourself when you keep at it. Make yourself a top ten list of all the other reasons you like moving your body and being fit, and read it often. The most important thing to remember is: Don't give up! Ever!

Hotels have been on the fitness bandwagon for quite some time, providing exercise equipment free or at a nominal fee to their traveling guest. Now airports are rising to the demand. With long delays, long layovers and odd arrival times irritating frequent flyers, a large number of airports in major cities and airline hubs have seen the wisdom of making arrangements with nearby fitness centers and health clubs for reasonable day rates. The health clubs have responded by keeping rates reasonable (in most cases) and even providing shuttles. For those without shuttles, the closest fitness center is usually only a quick cab ride away. Some airports even have workout facilities right on the premises!

A web site called airportgyms.com lets flyers type in a destination city and call up the workout possibilities available. On the list are health clubs in Baltimore, New York City, Chicago, Cleveland, Dallas, Los Angeles and New Orleans, to name just a few. In Chicago's O'Hare, Pittsburgh International, Las Vegas' McCarran and Miami International, workout facilities are right in the airport. In other cities, health clubs are a free shuttle ride or 5 to 25-minute taxi ride away. Day rates range from free--at the Bally's near Dallas/Fort Worth--to $15 at most participating airports. In Honolulu and New York's LaGuardia the nearest clubs charge $20 ($5 per hour at LaGuardia) and it's $25 at both airports in Washington, D.C.. But it sure beats sitting endlessly at the gate to see if your flight has been canceled.

Take Home Point: The one time you can become argumentative is when you feel an excuse not to exercise coming on. Debate your excuses and guard your workout time jealously. Do what you enjoy, vary your routine and chart your progress. Start simple and don't expect instant results. Just do it and don't quit.

Chapter 9: Five Ways To Get Moving - Fifty Ways To Keep Moving

A health club, exercise machines, aerobics routines and even a walking, running or jogging regimen are great ways to become fit, increase stamina, gain strength and burn calories. But they aren't the only ways to work out.

To overcome the inertia of a sedentary lifestyle and begin to enjoy the sensation of moving your muscles, a more gradual approach which increases your desire to exercise--your motivation--as it hones your ability, might be the best way to begin. One way to start is to identify those parts of your regular day that you'd consider "inactive," reduce them and replace with movement, gradually adding more intensity and activity as you go along. You can do this the most easily by exercise that doesn't feel like a workout, or by approaching your workout time in a different frame of mind.

Here are five ways to get yourself to begin exercising and 50 more ways to create movement and gradually begin working up to a more rigorous routine. They also work if you've stopped exercising for a period of time, if you find yourself in a slump or going through a hectic time where regular workouts just aren't possible.

Five techniques to get yourself moving:

1. Make a date with yourself: Write down your exercise time on your calendar or daily schedule--even if you're only going for a walk. Don't pencil it in, write it in ink and treat it as if it were an important meeting that you just can't cancel.
2. Make a date: Get a friend or partner to work out with you, or make an appointment with a personal trainer.

It's much harder to disappoint a friend or professional who has set aside a specific time for you than it is to cancel on yourself.

3. Work off a bad day or a bad mood: Treat exercise as a stress-reducer or a pressure relief valve. Vent frustration on the weight machines, the kickboxing class or with a high-intensity jog or run. Think of every single thing that irritates you and release it through your workout.
4. Fool yourself: Tell yourself you'll only exercise for 15 minutes; then you can stop. You might get caught up in the workout and forget all about the time.
5. Get steamed: Reward your workout by enjoying the other amenities of a health club or your own bath. Schedule a massage, hang out in the Jacuzzi or relax your muscles in the sauna or steam room. Luxuriate in a hot steamy bath or shower with your favorite music, scented candles and the best soap you can afford. Turn up the music and sing at the top of your lungs. You've earned some enjoyment.

And now, 50 ways to keep moving:

1. Take the stairs.
2. Park farther away and walk more.
3. On buses, subways or taxis, get off before your stop and walk.
4. Take a walk instead of a coffee break.
5. Start an exercise hour where you work.
6. Take up gardening.
7. Turn off the TV and move around from room to room.
8. Put on some music and dance.
9. Buy an exercise video and then use it.
10. Go to your co-worker's offices rather than using e-mail or the phone.
11. Rake the leaves into piles and jump into them, then rake them again.

12. Mow the lawn with a manual push mower.
13. Shovel the snow from your driveway and then your neighbor's.
14. Vacuum the entire house.
15. Clean out the closets or the garage.
16. Rent a carpet steamer and do it yourself.
17. Wash all your windows.
18. Jump rope or jog while watching TV.
19. If you work in an office, get rid of your chair and make phone calls standing up.
20. Play catch, Frisbee, tag or touch football withthe kids.
21. Play miniature golf.
22. On the real greens, don't use a golf cart.
23. Go bowling.
24. Weed the garden.
25. Wash all the floors.
26. Chop firewood, or at least stack it up by the fireplace.
27. Join the mall walkers, or go power-shopping.
28. Buy groceries at those big warehouse discounters and pack your own bags.
29. Scrub the kitchen and bathroom by hand.
30. Take dance lessons.
31. Shoot some hoops.
32. Take the kids (or grandkids) to the park and push them on the swings.
33. Go horseback riding--preferably at sunset.
34. Try snow-shoeing or cross-country skiing.
35. Walk the dog, or take it for a run.
36. Join a volleyball league.
37. Find a swimming pool and splash around like a kid.
38. Buy a Styrofoam "noodle" and take it into the pool, riding it like a horse.
39. Paint the house.
40. Help a friend move.
41. Go backpacking.
42. Row, row, row your boat, or canoe or kayak.
43. Re-arrange the furniture in all your rooms.

44. Hold a family picnic and have relay races, three-legged potato sack, tug-of-war, play badminton.
45. Take a petition for a worthy cause around your neighborhood for signatures--on foot.
46. Buy a bicycle, new or used, and feel like a kid again.
47. Wash and wax your car.
48. Go fly-fishing.
49. Pick your own fruits and vegetables on U-Pick-It Farms.
50. Go square dancing.

Take Home Point: Even exercise doesn't have to feel like exercise if you gradually replace sedentary activities with ones that involve more movement. Many enjoyable past- times can become the motivation for getting--and staying--in shape.

Chapter 10: One Thing of Which You Hardly Ever Get Enough

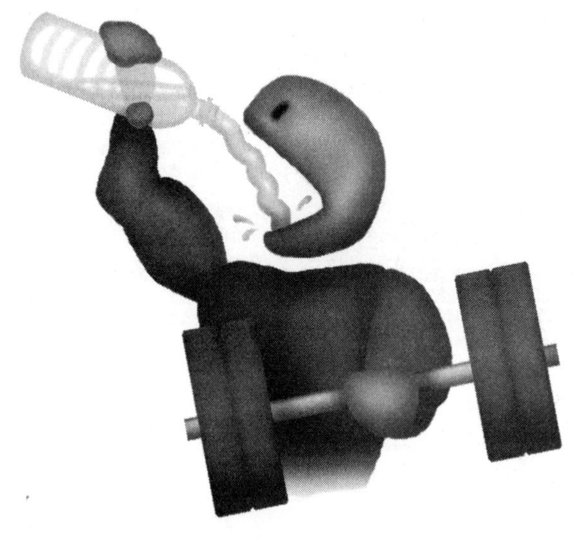

There's a miraculous substance that can aid any fitness plan, is good for your skin, can lessen your appetite, restore your energy and let you work and play harder. And it's usually free and without a single calorie. Want some of this miracle elixir? Turn on your tap! It's good old H2O.

In much of the world, good, clean drinking water is considered a luxury. But western civilization has been blessed with drinkable water in almost every city and town. So what do we do? We head down to the convenience store and plunk down a dollar or more for special drinks containing sugar and, at times, caffeine. Yet, as far as our mostly-fluid body is concerned, nothing beats good, plain old drinking water. You can, of course, spend money at that same convenience store for a bottle of water drawn from a special spring somewhere on the other side of the world. But most bottled water brands are nothing more than water drawn from municipal water supplies in some town or city in this country, then sold under a special brand name. Unless your region's drinking water is heavily chlorinated or the pipes are bad, turning on the tap at your kitchen sink and filling up a glass is as good as nearly anything you can buy. If you're really concerned, you can fill up a pitcher and leave it in the refrigerator overnight, or use one of the filtered systems on the market today.

The important thing is to drink enough water to avoid dehydration. Dehydration causes fatigue. By the time your brain tells you you're thirsty, you have already lost 1% of your body weight in water. At 2%, your performance decreases 10%. So, obviously, you shouldn't wait until you're thirsty to grab a drink because, by then, you are already dehydrating.

According to the American College of Sports Medicine, you should drink about a pint (16 ounces) of water before any physical activity. Then you should drink another 8-16 ounces about 15 minutes prior to the activity and at least 4-8 ounces every 15 minutes during the activity. You should even drink after you slow down again. A mouthful of water equals about one fluid ounce. And if you're hot, drinking water will do more to cool you off than pouring it over your head.

If you're competing in a sport, caffeine isn't a good idea. Water is still the best thirst quencher anywhere, anytime. Sports drinks contain sodium--salt--which insures that you're getting enough fluids into your body.

There's one other way water can help, especially if you're trying to lose weight. If you're feeling hungry, before you grab a snack, drink 8-16 ounces of water. Then, if you're still hungry, go ahead and eat. Sometimes thirst masquerades as hunger and, when you think you're hungry, your body is really just thirsty. At any rate, after you drink, you'll feel full enough to not overeat.

You would think that the most obvious failure to keep sufficiently hydrated would take place in desert climates, but American doctors have learned a lot about our own inability to ingest enough water, even at Arctic and Antarctic bases. Because of the cold, soldiers stationed in those places did not feel thirsty, would not drink enough fluids and would often suffer the effects of progressive dehydration, such as fatigue. Finally, they were urged to drink water at each meal, whether they were thirsty or not, and their symptoms disappeared. You must drink whenever you are thirsty, and always drink enough to saturate your thirst--or more. The experts notice that we often stop drinking water once our initial thirst is quenched, but that may not actually be enough to sufficiently hydrate our bodies.

Take Home Point: You need lots of fluids to keep from being dehydrated. Once you feel thirsty, it is already too late. Drink at least eight (8) ounce glasses of water or fluids other than alcohol each day or, if you are engaging in sports or physical activity, more thirst can also mask itself as hunger--so drink water first.

Chapter 11:
The Psychology of It All

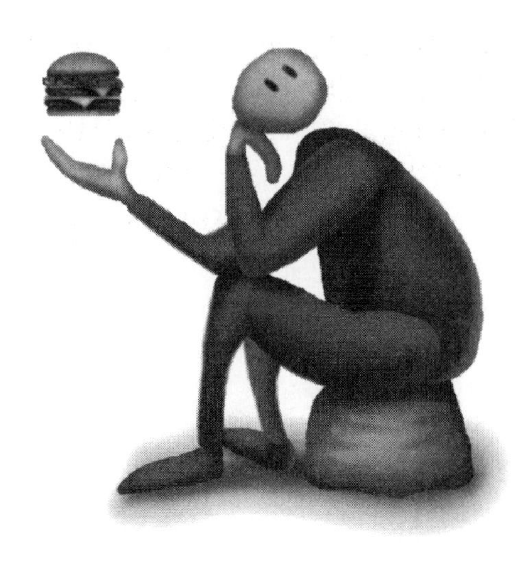

"It can't be this good," you're saying. "Something has to trip me up. There's got to be a down side."

You're right. Life isn't perfect, not everybody loves us, and when things seem all wrong, when you're angry with someone, when you're fearful, when you're lonely, it's only human to turn nearby to the one ready answer: FOOD! The more self-indulgent the choice, like something really sweet or salty, the better. It's just sooooo comforting to treat yourself and eat, at the time. And so discomforting later on when you realize what you've done.

If you feel unloved, you can at least love yourself with some food. Comfort and love. When the need for comfort and/or love becomes urgent enough, food is lying in wait to torpedo your plan. But, of course, food isn't a substitute for comfort. Food isn't a substitute for love. When something's bothering you and you're careless or unhappy, eating for the wrong reasons is a dreadfully poor choice to relieve the pain because it never does. It adds to the pain. And as for love? You're never going to find it by breaking your eating plan. In fact, you'll hate yourself afterward. It may be necessary to seek short-term counseling to help you work more directly with your feelings.

If eating for comfort or love is your habit, sure, it takes will to break a habit. But if you promise yourself at the outset, "My goal is eating for nourishment, and for the rightful satisfaction of eating," you'll eat the right things, in the right servings, at the right time.

Now, we come to the issue of size of portions, and the time-honored traditions of "seconds" and "thirds." A good healthy instinct, like eating when you are hungry, can become a self-destructive habit when it's eating when you're not hungry. For example, bingeing is an ancient custom. Actually, it's one of the seven deadly sins: gluttony. The Romans made an art of it -- especially certain of the emperors, and they were always the ones who died young.

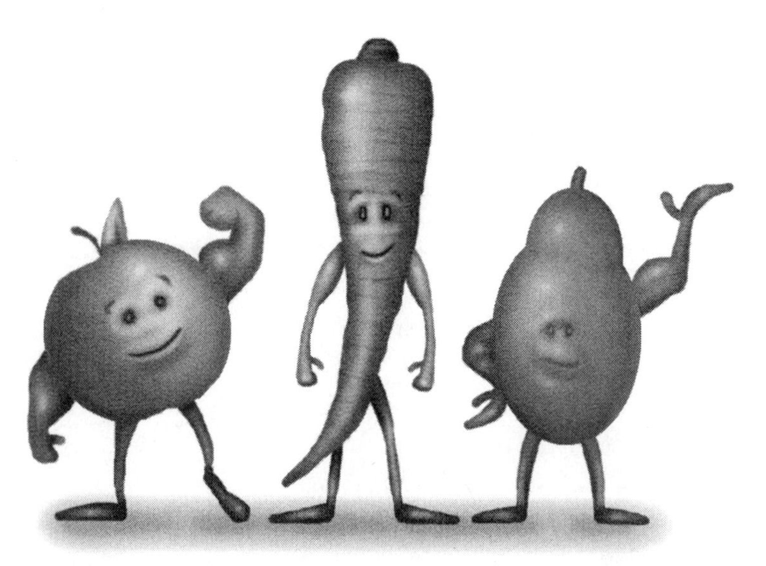

Finally, almost everybody has "trigger foods" that lead to overeating. Like eating for comfort or eating for love, eating trigger foods is addictive. You always want more and, once the trigger plate is removed, you want to eat anything. These foods lead right down the path to more, more, more. You have to identify what your trigger foods are, and not bring them home!

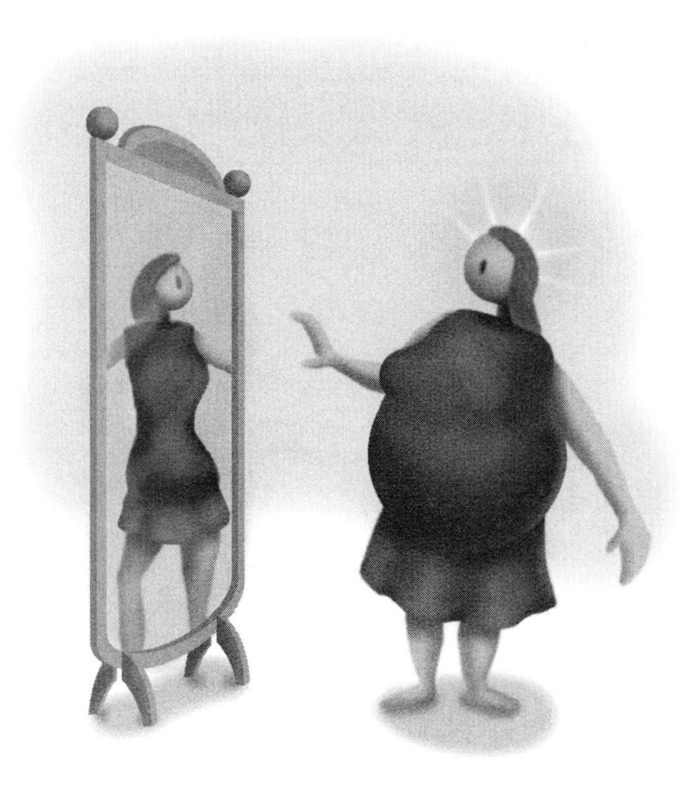

How do you see yourself? What is your body self-image? What would you like to see in the mirror? Rather than admiring some magazine or Internet image, how about making yourself as you would like to see yourself, your body image? That's the key, accepting who you are in the first place, maybe not exactly as you are right now, but as you see yourself after applying the principles, the techniques and positive attitudes gained in TOMORROW'S WEIGH®.

Take Home Point: We tend to eat for many more reasons than just being hungry. Try to identify what emotions or feelings prompt you to eat.

Chapter 12: Sometimes It Is All In Your Head

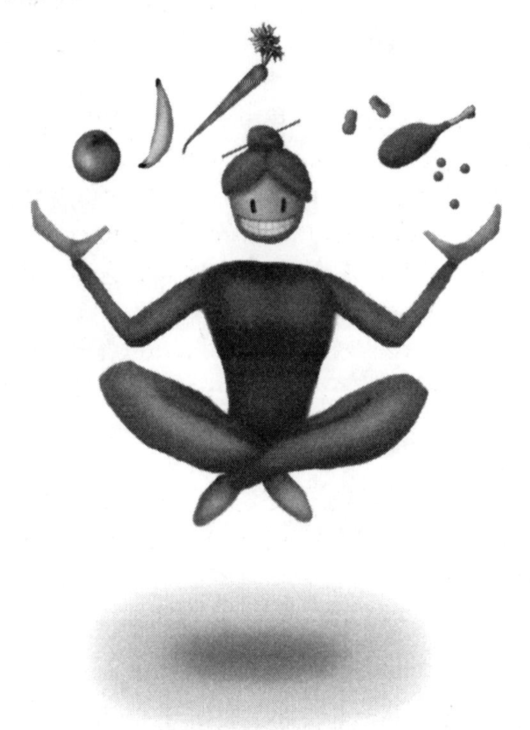

Knowing what to eat and finding ways to be more active are only the beginning steps to greater health and fitness and, ultimately, to long term weight management. Life is going to interfere; the best intentions are going to fall prey to stressful circumstances, and what's more important than any one menu or workout plan are the long-term strategies you'll choose in order to stick with a plan through the boring days and times when nothing seems to go as planned.

Psyching yourself up to stay on goal; uncovering the underlying reasons why you may get in your own way; identifying the pitfalls; and recovering from setbacks without resorting to self-blame and the "guilt-trap" are the mental and emotional tools necessary for any successful health program. It starts with self-knowledge which travels along the motivation path and leads to behavior modification that results in success. Part of this process is how you define success. You can't achieve your goals if you don't know what they are. Even if you carefully define exactly what you want to accomplish, you'll set yourself up for failure if you resort to perfection or define your acceptable outcomes too narrowly.

The first step is to figure out exactly what you're trying to achieve. Do you want to lose ten pounds? Reduce your intake of high fat foods or empty sweet calories? Avoid food binges? Get more fit or stronger? Reduce cholesterol? This is the stage where many weight loss plans head down the road toward failure before they even begin.

Experts in motivation and goal-setting have certain tried and true strategies to help build success into whatever new programs you undertake. To end up successful, they recommend that your goals:

• Be realistic: A 53-year old woman who has battled obesity all her life is setting herself up for failure if she wants to look like an 18-year old supermodel in six months. A better focus would be to target small weight-loss increments over a longer period of time and begin to work on bringing out her own personal best features. Tuning out the cultural messages of a youth-and-sex-obsessed media might be a required part of her goal-setting.

• Be measurable: Getting in shape means different things to different people and at different ages. Cutting your fat intake by 5% is a measurable goal. So is working out for 30 minutes three times a week.

• Start small and increase gradually: You shouldn't run a marathon if you've never even walked around the block. The same is true for weight loss. If that special event is six weeks away, you'll only frustrate yourself if you want to lose 100 lbs. by then. Small changes over longer periods of time spell success.

• Be re-evaluated as you go along: When you weigh 225 pounds, your calorie needs are greater than if you drop 30 pounds. Lifting 5 lb. weights for 15 reps is a good starting point, but you'll want to increase the intensity as you get stronger.

• Be rewarded: Celebrate your victories along the way by treating yourself to some special luxury or reward.

• Be written down: A goal that isn't written down is just a good idea. Those who write down what they want to achieve and review them often are more likely to succeed than those who just carry around a vague notion for improvement.

Health theorists have defined five stages of change which they say are required for success in behavior modification. When they tailored nutrition messages individually to suit a particular stage, they were successful in getting participants in a study to reduce their fat intake by 23% as compared with only 3% in a control group. The five stages are: pre-contemplation, when someone is unaware of a problem or the need for any change; contemplation, when they think about making changes in the near future; preparation, when a person actually plans to change; action, which means implementing a plan for change; and maintenance, which is the continuation of those actions over a period of time. In the pre-contemplation stage, a person may have to be made aware of the risks of an unhealthy diet or sedentary lifestyle, while the action and maintenance stages require support and rewards for someone to keep pressing on towards success. In attempts to get study participants to reduce fat in their diets, researchers found that only when they also targeted those in the maintenance stage, as well as the earlier stages, would such efforts reap success.

Take-Home Point: Goal-setting is an important first step to any health/weight management program involving fitness and health. Goals need to be realistic and measurable in order to succeed, as well as targeting both the long and short term.

Chapter 13: Tackling Triggers And Binges

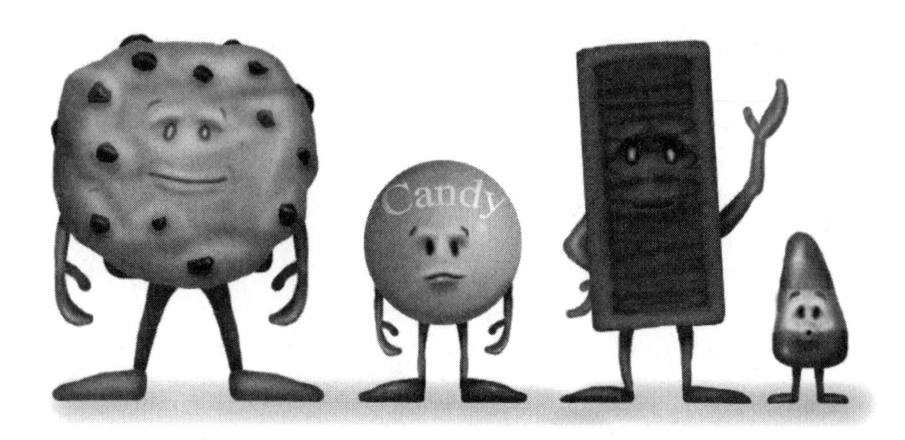

"Bet you can't eat just one," said the ad for a well-known brand of potato chip. In your case, you can pass up potato chips with no problem at all, but faced with M&Ms, you won't stop at just one bag. Are Oreos your downfall and you can't just buy two and satisfy a small craving? They're known as trigger foods, and figuring out your strategy before they are staring at you across the party table is key to sticking with your healthier eating plan over the long haul. But triggers are only part of the problem.

Cravings often lead to binges. Binges lead to guilt and guilt can lead you right back into overeating, setting off a vicious cycle that causes many well-intentioned self-improvers to throw out the entire plan and give up, figuring they'll never be strong enough to overcome such an overwhelming sequence of circumstances. We're not addressing severe food disorders such as bulimia here, just the inability to control eating that we all lapse into now and then.

Anticipating each stage of this downward spiral and fighting back with a well-planned strategy can take the power out of a binge, take the guilt out of a relapse and get you back on track without a big blow to self-esteem.

First, remember what we've said before about the eating and food choices. To avoid the guilt trap, it's essential to stop thinking about foods as either bad or good, to eat enough to sate your hunger and to incorporate sweets and treats into a well-balanced diet.

But what about those "trigger" foods? What happens when you go to sleep dreaming of chocolate chip cookies? Strategy number one is to identify your triggers so that they don't catch you off guard. What are those foods that you absolutely can't just eat a small amount of? Make a list and decide how you're going to handle it the next time you see them everywhere you turn. How about going to one of those mini-marts and buying only a small amount, even though you'll end up paying a lot more than at the mega-mart? Maybe you can share a bag with friends or co-workers, or go out to eat and order just a single serving. You might have to avoid your triggers completely, or save them for special occasions. Most people don't like to waste food, but rather than eating an entire bag of cookies or chips, or whatever your trigger happens to be, throwing out even a mostly full package (or giving it away) might be preferable to sabotaging your own efforts at healthier eating. As you diffuse your triggers, you might find that you can allow yourself a small amount to satisfy a craving without overdoing it.

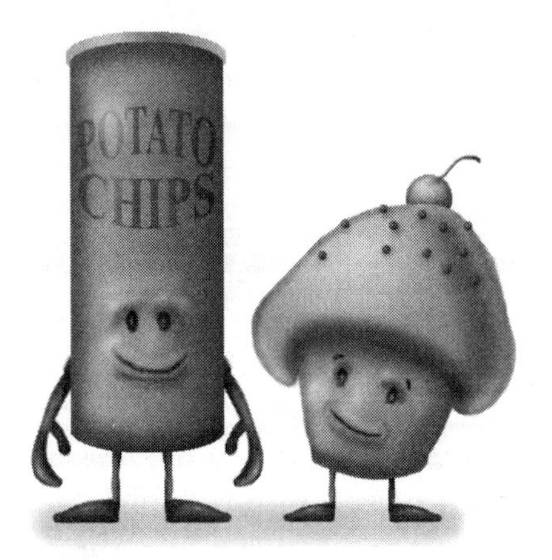

If you succumb to a binge attack, the first thing you need to do is take some sort of immediate or intervening action. Get up, walk around, call a friend, do whatever will put you on a different track right away. Two things you should not do are punish or berate yourself or feel excessive guilt. Put it into perspective–it's a minor setback, not the end of the world.

For the longer term, it helps to identify not only the "what" of trigger situations, but the where, when and why, as well as the how. Are there particular places, public or private, homes, parties, restaurant buffets--that trigger uncontrolled eating? Are you prone to binge in a certain mood, after a stressful day, only around the holidays or when you're feeling lonely? And what is your particular style of over-eating? "Picker/Nibblers" just pick endlessly while watching TV; "Prowlers" munch all day long; "Hoarders" eat very little until they are off by themselves, while "Finishers" clean every morsel from their plate.

The more you can bring food triggers and food bingeing into your conscious awareness, the more you can devise and execute a plan for keeping them out of your life.

Food bingeing may be our legacy from the days of the caveman, according to one psychotherapist with an online book. In Be Your Own Therapist, Thayer White notes that back in the days when we were hunter-gatherers, we had to take advantage of seasonal offerings and were likely to over-indulge in whatever was ripe at particular times of the year. If only we'd kept it to fruit! Thayer suggests that one strategy for dealing with uncontrolled eating of a particular food is to go ahead and have a planned binge. First, be especially careful to eat a healthy balance of nutritional foods most of the day. Then enjoy your craving, be it butter-cream frosting or, in his case, fruitcake! If you've already consumed enough foods high in nutrition and satisfied your normal hunger, you may end up self-regulating after only a small amount of your trigger foods. But even if you don't, you may actually grow weary of the food and it may lose its allure once you've taken away the seductiveness of the taboo.

Take-Home Point: Write down and become aware of foods, times of the day, places, feelings and life circumstances that trigger uncontrolled eating in your life, as well as your particular style of food bingeing. The more you plan and anticipate, the more successful you will be in maintaining a balanced eating plan.

Chapter 14: Find a Partner, a Support Team or Both

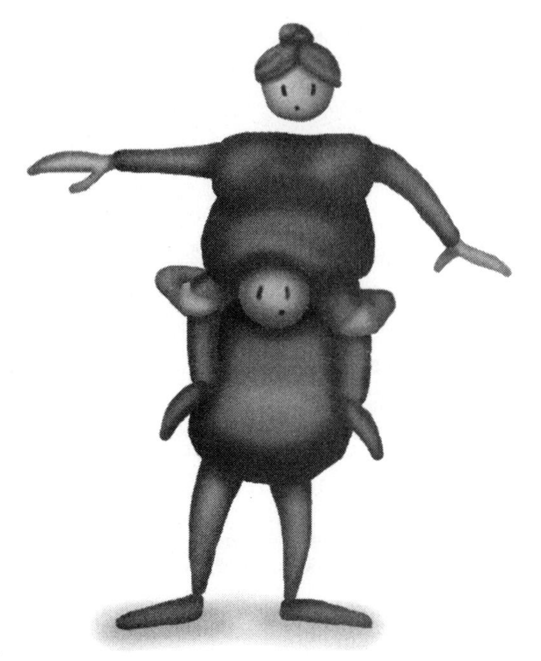

It's always easier to follow a food or exercise program by doing it with others. If going to the gym is an opportunity to "get together with the gang," have some laughs, or share some gossip, you'll have another reason to go. Best is to find a special someone as a training partner. Some of us find a physical trainer and pay a fee to have them motivate, advise, and make sure we're doing it all safely and in good form.

Even if you're home, about to do your stretching and aerobics or use your home gym, bringing a partner into it will make it better. You can count for each other, advise each other, and watch for one another's safety.

As far as preparing food or eating out is concerned, find someone to share it with, in the kitchen, over the phone, e-mail or fax with menus, or over the table.

It's wise to check in with some of the more formal means of support. Qualified private nutrition counseling will assure that you have a program especially designed for you. But beware of the faddist who tells you not to eat this or drink that. As previously stated about fad diets, faddist counselors can be dangerous to your health!

Make mealtime as exciting as a trip abroad. When you get bored with your menu, take a new perspective. The charts in our website, www.medicalnutritionconsulting.com are only suggestions. You can also get creative. Most ethnic foods such as Oriental, Indian, Caribbean, when fresh and well-prepared, are healthy and wholesome. National dishes from Spain, Portugal, France, Scandinavia, Greece, Turkey are adventurous and scrumptious too! Try and taste!

When exercises get really tedious, you'll discover as many varieties of aerobics, Tai Chai, JuJitsu, stretching and weight training as you can image.

So eat when you're hungry, enjoy the fresh air and deep breathing of exercise, and above all enjoy being yourself! That's TOMORROW'S WEIGH®!

Take Home Point: Find a friend or family member whom you trust to support you in reaching a healthy weight.

Chapter 15: When All Else Fails: Drugs or "The Knife"

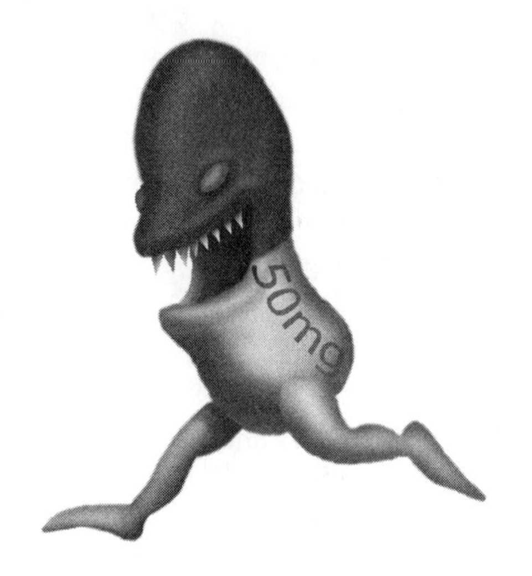

These two risky weight-management techniques are medically known as "pharma-cology" and "surgery". But "Drugs and the Knife" really say it better. ***

Drugs:

All drugs can be dangerous. We all know that. But worse, many of the weight-loss concoctions being peddled over the counter are not even approved and may be life-threatening.

Today's available drugs are another story. Or are they? At the time of this writing, the only two FDA-Approved as medically safe are Meridia and Xenical. Before we tell you of the risks or side effects and frequent lack of effect of these approved drugs, we warn of all the products out there that are NOT FDA-Approved medically safe. And there are more every day. They include: Callegen Nite-Loss Ultra, Fat Eliminator, Carbolock Rx and many more.

Meridia is known to cause dry mouth, sedation, and, in some cases, severe high blood pressure. However, it has achieved weight loss in some patients, actually only 30% of users lost 10% or more of their body weight.

Xenical causes 7 out of 10 to have abdominal cramps and flatulence (farting), along with diarrhea spotting their underclothes! However, it works. Those tested lost 9% of their body weight over six months.

Other drugs are legally available for limited use in certain patients: metformin, phenteramine and topiramate. Ask your doctor.

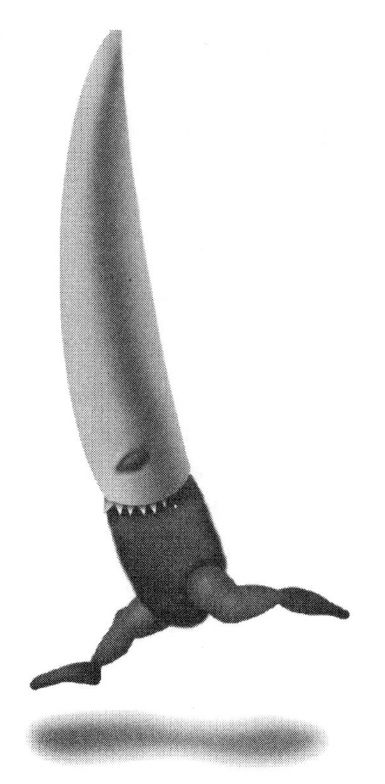

Can Surgery Help?

In a word, yes, if you follow the nutrition and exercise regimens recommended in this TOMORROW'S WEIGH® program. Forget liposuction and such. That just sucks out the fat from the surface and it comes right back.

The real problem is that your overweight body is insisting that you eat too much, so it can feed itself and stay like it is! One drastic option to solve that is surgery. It's drastic because - know this going in - all invasive surgery is risky. We don't care what it is. Don't go under the knife unless you absolutely have to. But-- that being said- if you are dangerously obese, you may have to! And it can change your body, and your life.

It's not your fault. It's instinctive! When there wasn't enough food all the time, the human body instinctively ate all it could, when it could, and stored the excess as fat for times when food was scarce! That's why it craves sugary, fatty, rich foods over healthy nutrition every time. Human nature!

But we don't live in a time and place when food is scarce, just the opposite. Here there's too much! And it's the wrong kind. It's what the food industry knows you crave-- junk food! And don't be fooled by "low fat" and "calorie free" because you NEED SOME FAT. And you're much worse off WITHOUT calories than with them!

If you are obese-- that is, a BMI of 30 or greater- your stomach has become permanently swollen. It demands the food to maintain itself and the rest of your heavy body. When you diet, you literally starve your body - never mind that you're too heavy. A swollen stomach, an over-overweight body demands more, more, more. As we said, it's instinct.

At some point, you have to consider "cut and paste". Your doctor will probably say when, but whether he does or doesn't, be sure to get a second opinion. Cut and paste is a lot easier on a computer than on the human body. What the surgeon will do, is install a gastric bypass. When you overeat, the food will bypass your stomach. Your stomach will shrink to normal size. You will want to eat less. You'll look better, feel better about yourself than ever before since you started to pile on the pounds.

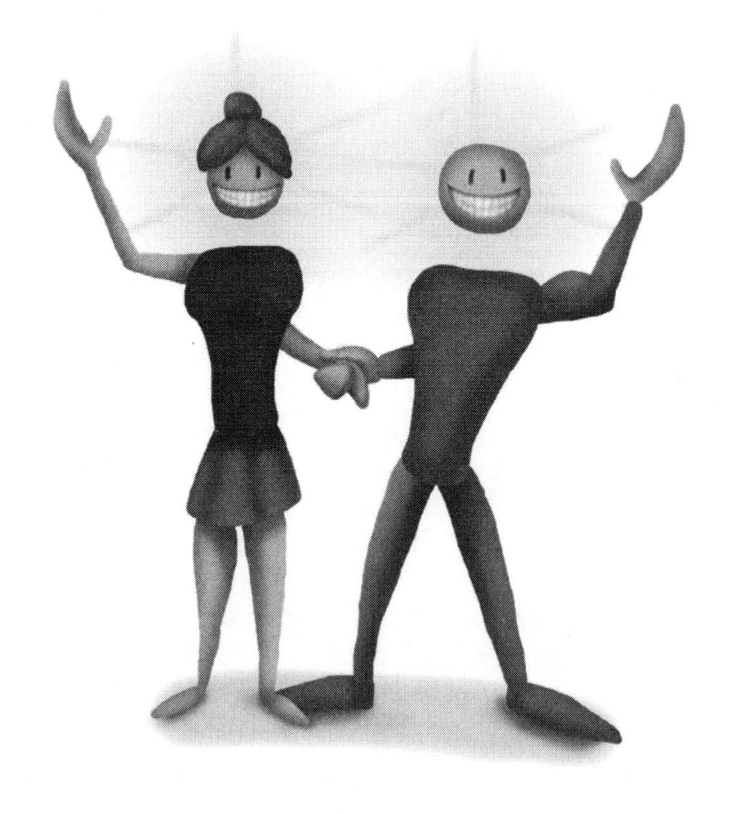

A Sorry History

The weight-loss drug craze began in the 1960's with the use of deadly "speed," that is, amphetamines. By the decade's end, we learned what many had known all along. They were addictive and had dangerous side effects. The practice of them was stopped. Then in the 80s, a doctor began getting results with "phen/fen." By 1996, two "magic cures" using Phen-fen reached the market and then Redux in 1997. Before long, the "magic" was over. The Mayo Clinic found phen/fen and Redux could cause valvular heart disease! Both were quickly taken off the market.

Take Home Point: In some cases, medications may be helpful in the treatment of obesity. Surgery is reserved for the morbidly obese where all of the attempts at weight loss have failed!

Chapter 16:

"Life entails courage; a life without courage ceases to be life."

-EM Foster

Diets are doomed to failure. They are a temporary fix to a much deeper problem. Your weight is simply a symptom of your disease process. Diets treat the symptoms. Tomorrow's weigh treats the root cause of the disease. If you had Strep Throat, would you expect to be treated only for your sore throat? What would happen if your doctor didn't give you an antibiotic? Actually we know what would happen. Your Strep Throat would lead to Rheumatic Fever and possibly death. This is the same disease process that is happening all across America with our weight. By only treating the symptom, namely weight, the disease process is proceeding into increased incidences of diabetes, heart disease, metabolic syndrome and hypertension, to name a few. If left untreated, these diseases will lead to heart attacks, strokes, amputations and death.

The reins are now in your hands…Do you have the courage to pick them up and change your lifestyle? We are here to help.

You begin with:

- Eating when you are hungry.
- Eating or drinking something for breakfast every day.
- Exercising daily.
- Identifying and controlling your intake of trigger foods.
- Eating proper portion sizes at regular intervals.

Wellness is more than just the absence of disease. A healthy lifestyle is the key to achieving wellness. The Tomorrow's weigh program promotes wellness, not weight loss.

Losing weight, as you know, is no easy endeavor. There is no quick fix or easy solution. But you can achieve your goal of weight loss with the Tomorrow's Weigh program. Thousands of people have lost weight and kept it off with this program, and you will too. That is because the weight loss becomes the new symptom of your lifestyle change, just as your weight gain was the symptom of your old lifestyle..

So, be courageous, turn the page and begin. If you become frustrated along the way, we are here: www.medicalnutritionconsulting.com. We offer on-line medical, nutritional and psychological support.

Learning Lifestyle Modifications
To Last
A Lifetime

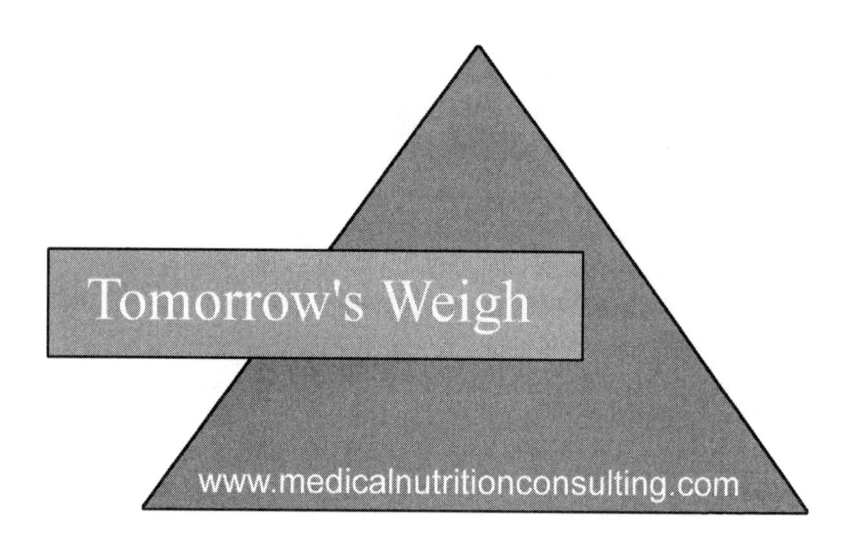

A special
Thank you
to
Debra Saltzman, LCSW
for her contributions to
Tomorrow's Weigh

Module One

Welcome! Congratulations on picking up the reins to your personal health. You have chosen the best possible program, and we are excited and looking forward to working with you as you achieve your personal goals.

You will be challenged by this program to let go of your beliefs about dieting and to begin to embrace a healthier, more realistic approach to managing your weight and health. This will be difficult at times and we encourage you to ask all the questions you have.

Housekeeping chores:

• Remember to plan at least one year to work through this program. Anytime shorter will not provide you with long term results.
• Whenever your life becomes chaotic and you find yourself not making the changes you had planned, DON'T QUIT! Too often, when we are doing well, we come to our sessions and when we are not doing very well, we stay away. If you are doing well and something comes up, well maybe it's ok to miss a session. BUT if you are not doing well, that is when you need to get to your session the most!
• Be sure to complete each module before going on to the next. It is hard to be patient, but you will need the tools from each module to completely work through the next.
• Email us with any question.
• This program will address how to eat, how much to eat, when to eat and why we eat. We will start with looking at our beliefs about eating and then move into planning our intake based on individual need. We will be looking at portion sizes, calorie needs, protein needs, fat needs, carbohydrate needs, exercise needs, hurdles that get in our way, and MORE!!

Before we begin, sit back in your chair for a moment and close your eyes. See yourself deleting all the beliefs you have previously had regarding eating, dieting, exercise and weight. Visualize that your mind as a clean floor, on which we are going to build some new ideas. Gone are the notions of good and bad foods. Gone are the notions that certain foods shouldn't be eaten or that you are bad if you do eat them. Gone is the notion that we are supposed to diet all day and still stay in control of our eating at night. Gone is the notion that life begins once we reach our weight goal.

Picture yourself in this big empty room and you are about to begin building a whole new interior. Each time you hear yourself saying, "Yes, but... stop and ask yourself, "What are you finding difficult to accept and why?"

Let's begin.

Travel back to kindergarten. Think about it. The human body has not made any updates in at least 30,000 years. That means that it has been using the same nutrients for all those years to keep the body alive and healthy. The body does not mutate very quickly! In fact, modern technology has us moving almost as fast as the speed of light, but our bodies are still in the neanderthol era!!

Current diets require us to believe that somehow, in a very short period of time, our bodies have changed. One year we no longer require carbohydrates and then, lo and behold in another year, we don't need any fats. Then, before we know it, we are told we don't need carbohydrates again! Whew.....no wonder people are sitting in America wondering what they are supposed to eat and not eat and decide, "What the heck" and leave for the buffet.

Let's go back to what we know to be true, based on science and what you learned in school.

There are six basic nutrient groups. They are carbohydrates, proteins, fats, vitamins, minerals and water. In order to be healthy, the body needs all six of these nutrients in their correct balance. It is just like a car. The car needs gasoline, transmission fluid, brake fluid, oil, water and antifreeze, but not all in the same amounts. If the car doesn't have gas, but has all the rest, it doesn't matter...it's not going to run. Like your body, your car needs all its "nutrients" in the correct balance.

Remember, a healthy diet is not about food, it's about the balance of nutrients. The dieting industry has placed all the focus on food and turned its back on nutrition. If you are seeking a healthy body and a healthy weight, then you need to place your focus on balanced nutrition.

Most people approach changing their diet with the concept that they must get rid of the "bad" foods and make up their new diets with "good" foods. Let's look at what most people consider "bad" and what most people consider "good."

Considered Bad	Considered Good
Desserts	Fruits
Chocolate	Vegetables
Ice cream	Chicken
Fast foods	Fish
Chips	Rice

The thought process is usually this, "I am not going to eat any more of the bad foods. I am going to clean out my house and my work place. From now on, I am going to eat only those foods that I know are good for me!" This usually lasts for maybe 1 – 4 weeks. And then what happens? That's right!! You can't stay away from the "bad" foods. Little by little or sometimes all at once, the bad foods start making their ways back into your diet. You become frustrated and finally throw in the towel, AGAIN!

Does it surprise you that this happens over and over again? It shouldn't, but, if you believed the diet industry, you bought into the concept that you should be able to control your eating regardless of the situation.

There are two false assumptions in the previous paragraph. The first is that you should be able to avoid some of your most favorite foods, forever. Well, that isn't going to happen. The most influential factor in how you eat is not your concern with health or weight issues, it is about "TASTE!" Taste will determine, in the long run, what you will be eating. If many of your favorite foods are on the "bad" list and you think you can avoid them indefinitely, you are setting yourself up to fail again. The second assumption is that foods are good and bad. Let's look a little closer at this. This is a hard concept to give up. Think about going to the grocery store and buying a bag of "good" foods and a bag of "bad" foods and then going and finding a chemistry room. Once in the chemistry room, you can perform an experiment that will prove our point. Take both bags of foods and break them down to their nutrient parts, which is what is done in the food laboratories for the food label information. When you are all done, all you will have as far as nutrients go, besides a mess, are carbohydrates, proteins, fats, vitamins, minerals and water……nothing else. This means that:

There is nothing nutritionally found in the "bad" foods that isn't found identically in the "good" foods. There is no such thing as a good or bad food.

There is only balance, just like the car! We need fats and carbohydrates just as much as we need proteins and vitamins. We just need it all balanced. This program will help you relearn what a balanced diet is. Or maybe, depending on your age, teach you for the first time.

Can your diet be balanced if all you eat are sweets, chips and fast foods? Of course not, but neither can it be balanced if you only eat fruits, vegetables and whole grains. To begin a healthy change in our eating patterns, we need a balance to the nutrients and to satisfy our unique tastes.

Each nutrient has a deficiency line and almost all nutrients have an upper tolerable limit. If any nutrient is taken in too low or too high a dose, there will ultimately be a negative outcome. For example, if you do not get enough iron in your diet, you will eventually become iron deficient and develop an anemia because the body can't make it. It relies on you to eat it. On the other had, if we get too much, our bodies will also become ill.

Think in terms of "balance," not "good or bad!"

Ok, if you have no questions or "yes, but's", then we will continue. Remember, if you have any questions, please e-mail us at www.medicalnutritionconsulting.com

Does it matter when I eat?

Absolutely!

Most of us have bought into the dieting industries message that we should be able to go all day eating very little and come home at the end of our day and be in full control of our eating. Yeah, right!

Think about how you usually feel when you come home at the end of the day. Do you come through the door and head straight to the cupboard or refrigerator? Most likely, especially if you were "good" that day and skipped breakfast and only had a light lunch. The diet industry has convinced us that we should go all day and eat as little as possible and then expect to stay in control of our eating when we get home. This will almost never work.

You body has certain physically "built in" regulators that will override the mind time and time again. Think about sleeping. Have you ever tried to stay awake for two days because you have so many things to finish? Do you find you can only go so far before your mind is still saying, "Stay awake", but your body says, "No way." You will go to sleep regardless of how much you want to stay awake. And, you can't sleep for only five minutes and get up and stay up for another 24 hours.

Your body will keep you asleep...like 5 – 7 hours!!

Let's look at another example: breathing. Can you hold your breath for five minutes? Of course not! It doesn't matter how conditioned you are, your body won't let you hold your breath for five minutes. If you can successfully hold your breath long enough, you will pass out and then, guess what? Right!! You will begin to breathe again!!

This is true with eating. Your body needs calories to stay alive, just like it needs air and sleep. If you try to withhold calories, you body will drive you to get the calories, just like it does with sleep and breath. You can't be expected to eat next to nothing and stay in control...your body won't let you. You will binge eat.

Once and for all, most of us need to give up those 1,000 and 1,200 calorie diets **forever**!!

Timing is everything, if you expect yourself to stay in control of your eating. Think about the last time you had your main meal mid-day. It may have been on a holiday or maybe on the weekend. See yourself on that day. Maybe your dinner was at 1:00pm or 3:00pm. Ask yourself, "How hungry were you at about 5:00pm or 6:00pm? You're saying, "I wasn't very hungry." That's because ironically, food is the number one appetite suppressant!! If you eat 2/3 of your intake by about 4:00 pm, you will find your hunger will decline as your day unwinds. You will make food choices according to your plan and you will feel better. You will also sleep better when your stomach is not full.

Step One

One of the first steps we need to take is to establish when we are going to eat, and then do it! Think about your work week and right now, establish a time for breakfast, lunch and dinner. Then think about your weekend and establish a time for breakfast, lunch and dinner.

Write down the times and then write down what you need to do in order to eat at those times. Do you have to plan your breakfast or make your lunch the night before? Do you need to have other people in your home take some of your responsibilities to free up some time? Do you need to let co-workers know that you won't be available for meetings at lunch? Try and think of as many hurdles that will prevent you form achieving this goal.

Don't worry about what you are eating yet, just get the timing down. You will be addressing what to eat later on. Remember, we will be working together for the next year.

Module Two

Review

How successful were you at following the times you have established for your meals and snacks?

How did you feel? Did you notice increased energy? bloating? sleepiness?

If you weren't able to adhere to the meal schedule that you had established, what got in your way? Are the obstacles movable? Does your schedule need to be modified?

If you have not been successful in eating at the times you set for yourself, please do not begin Module 2. Stay here and work on your timing. There may be other issues here that need to be addressed. One common issue is not being able to make time for yourself. This is a very big hurdle and one that needs to be behind you. If you can't seem to get around your hurdle on your own, the Tomorrow's Weigh team is here to help you. We are only a keyboard away!

Let's begin!

Once your meal and snack times are established, it will take continual effort to conform to them. You will be inclined to slip back to old eating habits when life gets chaotic. Keep working on it!

You must be asking; "What do we eat at these times? Where do we begin?"

We begin with the Food Guide Pyramid. The Food Guide Pyramid is a tool that was developed in the 1980's to help us insure a balanced meal plan. It was born out of the Four Basic Food Groups developed originally by Fredrick J. Stare, M.D., founder of the Nutrition Department at the Harvard School of Public Health.

There are different versions of the Food Guide Pyramid and include the Mediterranean Food Guide Pyramid, the Asian Food Guide Pyramid and the Vegetarian Food Guide Pyramid, to name a few. We will be working with the traditional Food Guide Pyramid, but you are encouraged to email us with questions if you follow one of the other versions. An updated version is due out in 2005.

As you can see, there are six areas identified in the pyramid. At the bottom is the Starch and Bread group. It is designed to comprise the base of our eating. We are encouraged to consume 6 – 11 servings daily. We will address what constitutes a serving shortly.

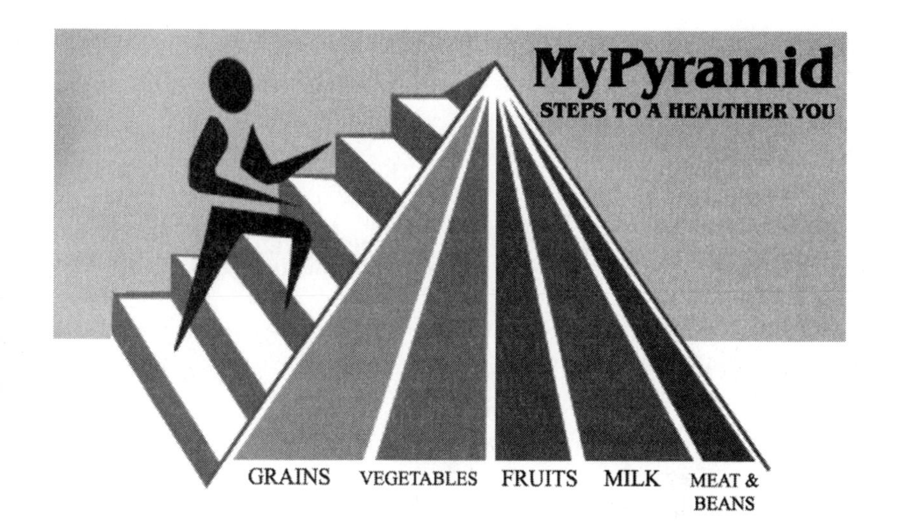

The next two groups are the Vegetables and Fruits. Vegetables require us to consume 3 – 5 servings and the fruits, 2 – 4 servings each day. All individuals are encouraged to Strive For Five, which is a total of five servings of fruits and vegetables combined.

The next two groups are the Dairy and Protein. If you are a grown adult, you need 2 –3 servings a day from the Dairy group and the equivalent of 4 – 9 oz of meat or meat substitute daily.

At the top of the pyramid are the Fats and Sugars. Keep in mind that Fats are vital for your health and provide essential fatty acids for proper cell development, that can't be made from anything else. You need a minimum of 3 fat exchanges daily.

But let's look closer at what is a serving. We'll start with the Starch group and work up the pyramid.

In the Starch group we find foods such as bagels, breads, cereals, starchy vegetables, crackers and rice. These servings sizes are taken from the Meal Exchange Booklet published by the American Dietetic Association and the American Diabetic Association.

Each serving in the Starch Group has approximately 80 calories, 15 grams of carbohydrates, 3 grams of protein and a trace of fat (less than 1 gram). The serving amount of each food in this group is based on these figures. For example, 1/3 cup of rice is a serving. That means that it has 80 calories, 15 grams of carbohydrate, 3 grams of protein and a trace of fat. If you have 1 cup of rice then you have eaten approximately 240 calories, 45 grams of carbohydrate, 9 grams of protein and a trace of fat. Let's look at other foods in the group and what amounts equal a serving.

Starch Group

Bread	1 slice	Pasta	1/3 cup
Bagel	1/4 piece	Rice	1/3 cup
Cereal	1/2 cup	Cooked Cereal	1/2 cup
Corn	1/2 cup	Peas	1/2 cup
Potato	1 small	Mashed potato	1/2 cup

In the Vegetable Group a serving is defined as the amount that contains approximately 25 calories, 5 grams of carbohydrate, 2 grams of protein and a trace of fat.

Vegetable Group (Non-starchy)

Raw	1 cup
Cooked	1/2 cup
Juice	1/2 cup

In the Fruit Group a serving is defined as the amount that contains approximately 60 calories and 15 grams of carbohydrates.

Fruit

Raw	Tennis ball size (Watch those soft-balls!)
Canned	1/2 cup
Dried	1/4 cup
Juice	1/2 cup

In the Dairy Group a serving is defined as the amount that contains approximately 90-150 calories depending on fat content, 12 grams of carbohydrate, 8 grams of protein and 0 – 8 grams of fat.

Dairy

Milk	1 cup
Yogurt	1 cup

In the Protein Group a serving is defined as the amount that contains approximately 25 – 75 calories, 7 grams of protein and 0 – 7 grams of fat.

Protein

Red Meat	1 ounce
Fish	1 ounce
Chicken	1 ounce
Tofu	1/2 cup
Beans	1/2 cup
Egg	1 whole
Egg White	2

In the Fat Group a serving is defined as the amount that contains approximately 45 calories and 5 grams of fat.

Fat

Monounsaturated	
Olive oil	1 teaspoon
Canola oil	1 teaspoon
Almonds	6 each
Polyunsaturated	
Corn oil	1 teaspoon
Margarine	1 teaspoon
Walnuts	6 halves
Saturated	
Butter	1 teaspoon
Lard	1 teaspoon
Shortening	1 teaspoon

The best place to look for the nutrition information in on the food label. Look and see how many calories and use that information to help you determine the portion that is appropriate for you.

Meal Planning

It is important to remember that everyone needs to consume the minimum servings from each group, each day. This will provide approximately 1300 – 1400 calories. Most of us will then need to add onto this base to bring us to the appropriate calorie range. This calorie range will be determined from your weekly food record. That is why it is so important that you report your intake as accurately as possible.

To begin to develop your meal plan, please find your Meal Planning Work Sheet at the end of this module. You will see that it is set up for three meals and snacks. Take out your weekly planner and determine what your schedule is for the week. Write in activities that are going to impact on your meals. For example, do you have a late night at work, a meeting in the evening, or the kids have practice from 6:00pm – 8:00pm.

Next, starting with your breakfast, write down what you plan on having. For example: Two pieces of whole grain toast with low-fat peanut butter, one small banana, a cup of coffee and 4oz of orange juice. Remember, after the whole day is planned, we should have the minimums from each food group represented. So, for breakfast we have: 2 starches, 2 fruits, and 1 fat. Now complete each breakfast for the rest of the week.

Do this same exercise for your lunches.

Now, for dinner, it is a little different. We will have to look at those activities and plan quick meals or meals that have been prepared ahead of time, for those evenings. Write in the meals you will be using. For example, does a stir-fry work on the night you have a meeting? A stir-fry can be completed in 20 minutes and provide a complete meal.

Write down all the protein sources that you use such as chicken, turkey, ham, beans, red meat, fish or tofu. Begin to write in the corner of each dinner block which protein source you will use on that day. Rotate the protein sources so that on Monday it is chicken, Tuesday it is red meat, Wednesday it is fish, Thursday it is meatless, etc. Once that is done, go back and decide which chicken dish you will make, which red meat dish you will make, etc.

At this point you should be looking at your meal planner and see that your breakfasts are filled in, your lunches are filled in and now your dinner's protein source is identified. If this is true, let's finish our meal plans for this week.

You will want to have a starch, dairy, vegetable and a fruit with the protein source. Here it is important to remember color. You want to have your meal be appealing to eye as well as to the mouth!

Let's work through a day. We'll pick a chicken day, as so many of us are using a lot of chicken.

We will bake our chicken in the oven. We will plan on an hour and fifteen minutes for the chicken to cook. Now, keeping in mind that chicken is basically white in color, we will want to pick other foods that have color. The starch group is usually also white, so it won't matter if we pick rice or potatoes or a noodle. We can jazz up the starch by cutting up a red or green pepper and making a confetti effect mix in, or just serve the starch as it is.

The vegetable and fruit selection will really bring your meal to life. Let's pick a bright green broccoli, a bright orange carrot or maybe a fresh salad with greens and reds and yellows. For the fruit, we can choose orange slices or a bunch of red grapes on the side of the plate, or maybe take a yogurt for your Dairy and mix a fruit in. These ideas only take a few minutes to prepare and will add brightness to your plate and nutrients to your body!

Now complete the rest of the week. Are you having problems? Please email us and let us help.

Finally, we have your snacks. Go back and review your days and compare them to the Food Guide Pyramid. What is missing? That should be your snack. If nothing is missing, you get to pick!!

Ok, let's reassess where we are.

We have our meal times and now we have our meal plans for the week. Last, we need the groceries. Make a list of all the foods that you don't have in your house. Add your staples to it, such as milk, bread and fruit and you are set to go shopping.

Working with a list will not only save you money, but also will limit the amount of impulsive buying for which the grocery stores are designed.

Step Two

Plan your meals for each week, or even in two-week intervals. Make up your grocery list to be sure you have what you need.

Review your meal times and be sure that are appropriate for your week.

E-mail us if you are having problems.

Tomorrow's Weigh
Meal Planning Work Sheet

	Breakfast	Lunch	Dinner	Snacks
Monday				
Tuesday				
Wednesday				
Thursday				
Friday				
Saturday				
Sunday				

Grocery List

Module Three

Review

How was your week? Did you stick to your times? Did you follow your meal plan? Did you find yourself with more energy? What were the obstacles that you experienced? Did the portion sizes surprise you? What were your portion sizes?

Let's Begin!

You are beginning to experience a new and healthier lifestyle. The changes will bring moments of new insights, as well as moments of disappointment. The important thought is to never quit.

You never fail unless you quit. Health is a life-long process that requires on-going attention. It is a process that you work with every day.

While you continue to work on timing and meal planning, we are going to take the next step into increased activity.

Many factors have played into the decreased activity experienced by Americans. Some of these factors include: community design with regional schools and urban sprawl; increased technology; increased fear of security; increasing numbers of automobiles; decreased biking/walking path availability; and school districts that are trying to balance budgets and, in the process, are eliminating physical education. Sixty years ago people used to cover approximately nine miles everyday in daily activities. We now cover an average of two!

A key factor in maintaining your metabolism is your percent of lean muscle. If you allow yourself to become increasing inactive, your lean muscle will begin to atrophy. You will also notice decreased stamina, increased fatigue, and decreased strength and flexibility. It is crucial to weight management that we all maintain our lean muscle.

You can lose weight without exercise, but keeping it off and trying to be healthy is another story.

Let's take a closer look at your physical activity. Starting with your daily routine, are you at work or are you at home? If you are at work, do you sit most of the day or are you up on your feet and moving? If you are at home, are you chasing children, or do you find yourself sitting and reading or listening to music or watching television?

The new guideline for **ALL** people is to be active, over and above your usual daily activities, for a total 30 minutes **every** day. This can be done all at once or accumulated throughout the day. If you have been inactive for a while, it is important to begin slowly and work up to the 30 minutes.

If 30 minutes seems to be a lot, think of it this way. Would 30 minutes of television be too much? Let's look closer at the dynamic of your exercise. There are two types of exercise: Aerobic and Anaerobic, also known as Cardio and Strength.

Aerobic or Cardio exercise is targeting the cardiovascular system and helping keep the health of the lungs, heart and blood vessels intact. It is also great at boosting the metabolism and burning body fat.

Anaerobic or Strength exercise is targeting our muscular system. Our muscles will atrophy when not used, as well as with the aging process. Strength training is responsible for maintaining our lean muscle and helping to boost our metabolism.

These two forms of exercise, when integrated together into an activity regime, will produce the best results.

Movement is not something we do only when we are focused on weight loss, but something that needs to be as second nature as brushing your teeth.

Before beginning any activity program it is necessary to check with your physician first and obtain a clean bill of health. Once that is in hand, another door just opened and it is guaranteed to bring you increased energy, improved quality of sleep, improved mood and a smile to your face!

Each individual has preferences for activity. Please take time now to determine which type of exercise you prefer. You may want to begin working with a personal trainer to establish a program that is tailored to your needs, limitations and goals. Or, you may want to begin with walking in your neighborhood. The important thing is to begin somewhere.

Please go to your physical activity record, located at the end of this module and begin tracking your progress.

We will continue to assess our progress as we proceed.

Before we leave, let's take a few minutes and explore the hurdles that have taken us off track in the past and those that might sideline us in the present and future. Please review chapters 8 and 9.

Excuses abound for not moving: I don't have time; it is too costly; I don't have anyone to do it with; I have bad ankles – knees – back; the weather is awful; I'm just too tired.

Remember, where there is a will, there is always a way.

Step Three

Take a moment and write down your current excuses. Look at them. If they really seem insurmountable, please e-mail us so we can help you move beyond them.

Activity Record

Goal:____

	Monday	Tuesday	Wednesday	Thursday	Friday	Saturday	Sunday
Week One							
Week Two							
Week Three							
Week Four							

Module Four

Triggers and Eating Cues

Review

How are you doing with your recording and meal planning? Are you finding that you are slipping back into old habits? Are you forgetting to go grocery shopping on a regular basis? Are you packing "meals on the run"?

How are you feeling after beginning your exercise routine? Are you enjoying the exercise? Do you have a partner, or do you prefer to exercise alone?

E-mail us if you are struggling, so we can coach you through the difficult times.

Let's Begin!

Remember that there are no "good" or "bad" foods. There are only the six nutrients, namely carbohydrates, proteins, fats, vitamins, minerals and fats. All food is made from these six nutrients. When taken to a chemistry lab and closely examined, there is nothing lurking in certain foods that is going to undermine your efforts!

Trigger foods

Sometimes you may find that, if a certain food (or foods) is in the house, it seems to call your name continually, until it is gone. These types of foods are almost exclusively carbohydrates. Foods such as potato chips, corn chips, ice cream, bread, certain kinds of cookies, pie or cake are a few examples of typical foods usually calling your name.

These foods are called, "Trigger Foods." They are not "good" or "bad", but rather particular foods to which you are sensitive. These foods are unique to you. It is important for you to recognize these foods and begin to realize the effect they have.

Take a moment to think about your trigger foods. Make a list of them, so that you are very aware of which foods they are. If you do not have any trigger foods, move on to the next section about behaviors.

My Trigger Foods

____

____

____

____

____

____

Usually we buy these foods under the disguise of having these foods available for our family or friends if they drop by. We will see these foods on sale, or sometimes visit a certain store because we know that they are sold there.

This is all very noble, but it is important to face your trigger foods and realize that you need to **stop** buying them and bringing them into your home.

Losing and managing weight has many positive outcomes. Most of us begin our weight loss program with great anticipation of feeling and looking better when we get to our weight goal. While it is true that we will feel and look better as we lose weight, too often we forget about the negative outcomes associated with weight loss and management. What could be negative?

Managing weight requires regular exercise. When you are not managing weight, you can easily tell yourself it doesn't matter if you exercise or not. If you chose to manage your weight, it always matters, and you don't have the luxury of not exercising.

Managing weight also means that you can't eat what you want, when you want, in any quantity you want. Managing weight means that you have to plan your meals, practice portion control and eat at generally the same time each day.

Trigger foods are usually your favorite foods. Obtaining and managing weight loss means that you will no longer be able to bring these foods freely into your environment, unless you have every intention of consuming all of it. There is no more "disguise" of having these foods around for family or friends. You need to remove them from your home.

Does this mean that you can never have them again? No, it doesn't. What it does mean, however is that you will need to purchase these foods only when you are out. You will need to purchase a predetermined amount and then eat and enjoy them.

Behavior Maps

Whenever we try to determine how to make our way to a new location, we frequently look at maps, or make our own. Our behaviors make a map that frequently leads us to the same destination time and time again. Let's look at an example given by a past participant.

Kate use to come home from work each day at approximately 5:30pm. She has two children who are active in sports. Depending on the evening, Kate would usually have to provide dinner, get the children to their activities and home again. She also had to be sure that they completed their homework, oversaw their baths and be sure their cloths were clean for the next day. Bedtime was usually at 9:00pm. Once the children were in bed, Kate would clean up around the house, get things ready for morning and then sit down in front of the television. Once in her favorite chair, Kate's thoughts frequently turned to what was there to eat in the kitchen. She almost always found herself eating, right before she went to bed.

Kate would wake up the next morning and tell herself that she wasn't going to eat that late again. This happened day after day.

Let's make a map of Kate's trip through the evening.

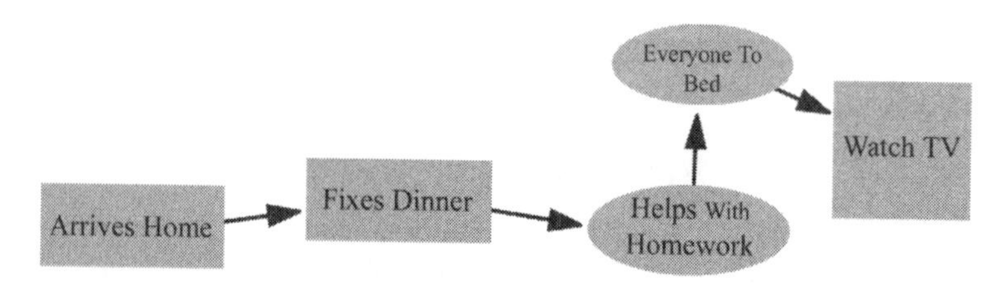

Once Kate has settled down to watch TV she immediately begins to think about what there is to eat in the kitchen.

Make your own map. Do you find that you travel the same trip each day and end up eating when you didn't intend to? Once you can observe your map, you can begin to re-route your trip. In Kate's case, her eating had become a reward for completing all her jobs and chores. She would relax and de-stress in front of the television. Her eating was part of the de-stressing. Once she saw the trip she made most evenings, she realized she could re-route her trip. Kate started going into another room at night, after all her work was done, and she read books and magazines that she enjoyed. She found that, by moving into another room, it was easier to stop her nighttime eating.

Think about other ways you can reach your destination, that doen't involve eating.

Step Four

Complete your trigger list and recognize the need to keep these foods out of your home.

Map out your trip that leads you to eating situations that are problematic for you. E-mail us if you have questions. We are here to help you create new habits to support your weight loss and maintenance.

Module Five

Review

Lifestyle changes take a lifetime to perfect. Don't get discouraged if you discover that changes you put in place a few weeks ago have somehow disappeared. Let's take a minute to review where we've come and what we have put in action.
Ask yourself these questions:

- Are you eating 2/3 of your intake by 4:00pm?
- Are you remembering to have snacks on hand for the morning and afternoon?
- Are you sticking with your exercise routine? If it isn't working, have you tried something new, or emailed us?
- Have you made a list of your trigger foods and realized the need to control when and where you have these foods?
- Have you made maps/paths of trips you take that lead you into unplanned eating?

If you need to go back to any of the completed modules, do it now because it is important to your success that you complete each step before going on to the next.

Let's begin

Going to the grocery store requires us to read food labels. The food label gives us the information we need to choose our foods and beverages wisely.

Go to your kitchen and pick a food with a food label and refer to it during this module.

The first item on the label to notice is the portion size. The portion size is the amount that reflects all the nutrition information. It is not necessarily the same amounts noted on the food pyramid. Also notice how many servings are in the package you are holding.

The next item is the calories. This is helpful when determining how many calories you are eating. Too often we consume larger amounts than we realize. The calories from fats are usually the grams of fat times 9. This information allows you to determine the percent of calories that are from fats.

Next on the label is the Total Fat. It is suggested that the healthy diet should have between 25%– 35% of calories from fats. This is up from the previously recommended amount of 30%. The majority of fat should come from Monounsaturated fat, which is found in olive oil, canola oil, peanut oil, almonds, avocados and walnuts. Saturated fat, which is from animals, should be minimized.

Saturated fats should make up no more that 7% of calories. The way to determine this is to multiply the total calories you consume on a daily basis by .07. For example, if you are losing weight and consuming approximately 1800 calories, then 1800 X .07 = 126 calories. Then, because all the information on the food label is in grams(gm) or milligrams(mg), we have to divide by 9. We divide by 9 because there are 9 calories per gram in fats. Therefore, the total saturated fats each day = 14 grams. Try determining the amount of saturated fat you should be having. Having difficulties, email us.

Next is sodium. When looking at this number, always given in milligrams(mg), it not unusual to wonder how much we should be eating. A no added salt (NAS) diet provides approximately 1,110mg to 3,000mg/ day. Use this number when assessing the amount of sodium in your diet. If you have high blood pressure or a family history of heart disease, you will want to keep your daily sodium intake in this range.

Next is Total Carbohydrate, followed by Fiber and Sugar. There is a lot of confusing information regarding the amount and type of carbohydrate we need. The current recommendations are to have between 45% – 60% of total calories from carbohydrates. Now remember that carbohydrates are found in starches such as breads, fruits, dairy and vegetables. They are also found in sweets and other snack type foods. The following table will let you look at where the carbohydrates, proteins and fats are found.

	Carbohydrates	Proteins	Fats
Starch	15gms	3gms	0-1gms
Fruit	15gms	0gms	0gms
Vegetable	5gms	2gms	0gms
Dairy	12gms	8gms	0-8gms
Meat	0gms	7gms	0–8gms
Fat	0gms	0gms	5gms

When determining the amount of carbohydrate you need in your diet, you need to ask yourself certain questions.

- Is there a family history of diabetes in your family, or do you have diabetes? If you answered yes to this question, you will want to keep total carbohydrate between 45-50% of calories.
- Do you participate in physical activity every day? If you answered yes to this question, you will want to keep total carbohydrate between 55-60% of calories. If you don't have diabetes in your family and you are not physically active, you will want to keep total carbohydrate at 50-55% of calories.

To determine the amount, let's use the same 1800 calorie example we used in determining fats. Take 1800 calories and multiply by .50 for 50% of calories. 1800 X .50 = 900calories. Now divide this number by 4, because there are 4 calories per gram of carbohydrate. 900/4 = 225gms. Try it with your calorie range.

Simple sugar should not exceed 10% and is calculated the same way, and is part of the total carbohydrate amount. 1800calories X .10 = 180 divided by 4 = 45gms. Therefore, of the total 225gms of carbohydrates a day, 45 can be from simple sugar.

Fiber should be between 20 – 35gms each day. Fiber has been shown to help maintain blood sugar levels, lower cholesterol, keep you feeling fuller longer, and possibly decrease the risk of GI cancer.

Protein needs to be between 12 – 20% of calories. It too is calculated the same way. If we use the 1800calories as an example, we need to multiply 1800 by .12 and .20.
1800 X .12 = 216/4 calories per gram = 54gms.
1800 X .20 = 360/4 calories per gram = 90gms.

Using the information on the food label can be very helpful, when determining the balance of your diet. If you have further questions, please email us.

Step Five

Determine the balance of carbohydrates, proteins and fats in your diet, based on the total amount of calories you are consuming. It will help you maintain a balance to your diet that will help prevent obesity and disease.

Module Six

Review

Life has a way of changing even the best-laid plans, so it is always important to go back and review whether you are still doing what you think you are doing.

Answer the following questions:

- •Are you planning and eating three meals daily? Yes_____ No_____
- •Are you planning your snacks daily? Yes_____ No_____
- •Is there protein in all your meals? Yes_____ No_____
- •Is your exercise done daily? Yes_____ No_____
- •Are you consuming 5 fruits/vegetables daily? Yes_____ No_____
- •Are you aware of portion sizes? Yes_____ No_____
- •Are you thinking in terms of good and bad? Yes_____ No_____

If you answered "No" to any of these questions, you need to go back and adjust your lifestyle so that you can then answer "Yes." Once you have answered "Yes" to all the questions, you are ready to proceed.

Let's Begin!

We are going to go on a virtual supermarket tour. There are a few things you will need to bring with you. Take a moment and get your meal plan for the next week. Be sure to check your cupboards, refrigerator and freezer for what you have on hand. Make a shopping list of the things you need to buy. Once you have your list, we are ready to go!

Before we go in, let's think about the layout of the grocery store. The perimeter of the store contains most of the products that have not been manipulated. They usually include the produce, meat, dairy and bread sections. You may not be able to find a food label on many of these foods, with the exception of the breads and some dairy products. The aisles usually contain the foods that have been manipulated, and almost all contain food labels. It will be in the aisles that you will find most of the additives and higher levels of sodium.

Entering the store, grab a cart and head to the Produce section. The produce section is where you will be purchasing the fruits and vegetables that you will need for the week. Remembering that we need 5 servings of fruits and vegetables daily will determine the amounts we need to purchase.

The reasons why fruits and vegetables are so important to our diets are many. They provide a wide variety of vitamins and minerals that help to maintain your vision, your bones, your heart and your nerves. The colors of the fruits and vegetables have been identified as providing vital immune enhancing/disease fighting strength to our bodies.

Remember, when selecting your fruits and vegetables, you will need to look for the brightest and deepest colors you can find. The richer the color, the more disease fighting power the fruits and vegetables have.

Pause for a moment and look around. What do you see? You should be seeing a whole array of colors, from bright greens to brilliant reds, vibrant oranges, beautiful yellows, and more. Capture this picture in you mind and, when you leave the produce section, your shopping cart should reflect this picture. Can you identify some fruits and vegetables that you have never consumed? Try buying just one, of a fruit or vegetable you've never eaten, each week. Little by little, you will expand your produce choices.

Moving on, we make our way into the **Meat** section. It is in this section where you find a rich supply of proteins, with their life building amino acids, iron and vitamin B-12. Let's separate this section into animal, fowl, fish and plant protein sources.

Before we begin, the quality of our protein is important to our health. We need to consume quality proteins if our bodies are going to be able to make all our cells properly. The perfect protein source is the egg. All other protein sources are compared with the egg to determine how good their amino acid blend is.

We'll start with the **Animal** section. Let's consider that all animals have a similar shape. The front and the back end of the animal is where you find most of the muscle. The cuts from these areas tend to be cheaper and leaner. They usually need to be slow cooked, with moist heat. The center of the animal is where you find the most tender and flavorful cuts, but also the extra fats. The center cut meats do not require manipulating, marinating or manually tenderizing.

The following will identify those meats that are the leanest, to those meats which have the highest fat content: USDA Select or Choice grades including round, sirloin, and flank to higher fat content grades like Prime, corned beef, shortribs, and meatloaf.

Moving on to the **Fowl** section, we find that this meat is very lean, and can be utilized in many recipes. White meat is always very lean, and, although the dark meat contains slightly more fat, it is still considered lean. Even wild fowl, like duck, is lean, as long as the skin is removed.

An interesting point is that wild meat is always lean, because the animal/fowl is always on the move. It is only the domesticated animal/fowl that is "fattened."

The following will identify the fowl cuts that are the leanest, to those that contain more fats: white meat of chicken and turkey without skin to higher fat choices like dark meat with skin, fried chicken with skin, or fatty ground chicken or turkey.

Moving on to the **Fish** section, we can enhance our intake of the heart-healthy, Omega-3 fatty acids.

Caution: Fish that traditionally weigh more than 20 pounds need to be consumed in limited amounts. Women who are pregnant should avoid eating fish that weigh more than 20 pounds, especially shark, sword, king tile and mackerel.

For many years, shellfish was considered high in cholesterol, and therefore, not good to eat. That thought has changed over the past 10 years, and now ALL fish is considered healthy to eat. It is suggested to consume fish three times weekly. If you don't like fish, but you would like to try and increase the amount you are consuming, try starting with some of the more mild flavored fish. You may also want to try to begin eating fish by ordering it when you are eating out. Many people struggle with ways to prepare fish, and also may not like the smell.

Last, but not least, we have the **Plant** section. We often forget the health benefit of consuming plant proteins. They are fairly low in calories, low in fats, high in fiber and have an abundance of vitamins and minerals.

Beans are one of the primary sources for plant proteins. There are many varieties of beans and they can be quite versatile. They go in soups, stir-fries, and salads, and the Italians have been making "pasta fagioli" for years. (translated, is pasta and beans.) At first, beans may cause an increase in flatulence, but that is only temporary, until your body gets used to them.

Soy is another excellent source of plant protein. All parts of the soybean have been used to make soymilk, tofu, yogurt, and have even been transformed into the shape of hamburgers and sausage!

Now we turn the corner and head to the cereal aisles. Have you ever noticed that the center shelves have the sweeter cereals on them?

Caution: Remember that even the grocery store is about "sales." Everything is arranged to entice you to spend money, right down to the end of the aisle displays and the checkout counters.

When trying to decide on the cereal you want, remember that there are no good or bad foods. Key things to get from your cereal include fiber, vitamins and minerals, and carbohydrates. Be sure to look at the portion size and the associated calories. Some of the cereals can be very high in calories, and you may want to choose another one.

Try to pick a cereal with at least 3 grams or greater of fiber. The vitamin/mineral content of most cereals is almost equal to taking a multivitamin/mineral supplement.

Caution: Remember that the more a product is manipulated, the less of the original nutrition content it contains.

If you are eating oatmeal for the cholesterol lower effect, you will need to use the slow-cook kind. Instant oatmeal is not effective in lowering cholesterol.

As you make your way through the aisles in the store, it will be important to call on the knowledge you now have in reading the food label. Watch your sodium, additive, and hydrogenated oil content.

In the **bread** section, you want to pick breads that contain at least 2 grams of fiber per slice. Many types of bread advertise as being multigrained, but when you look closer, you discover that there isn't much difference between them and white breads. If you find that you do not like the taste of the higher fiber breads, that is ok. You will just need to be more aware of getting your fiber from other foods.

Finally, in the **dairy** aisle, you will want to look for lower fat products that you like. If you are now drinking whole milk, don't try going to fat free, unless you really know that you will be able to learn to like it fairly quickly. Try going first to 2% and slowly bringing the fat content down. Anytime you find that you just don't like the taste of the lower fat products, try using less of the higher fat foods.

Step Six

Be sure to shop at least every two weeks. If the foods are not in your home, your eating plan is going to fall apart. You will not be able to maintain a healthy diet or a healthy weight.

Module Seven

It's week seven, and your motivation for making this major lifestyle change may be slowing down. We have found that, at this point in your transformation, many individuals state that their initial motivation has started to wane.

It is important that you realize that if your motivational level is changing, it is normal. Now is the time, however, to once again decide what it is that moves you toward making this healthy lifestlye change?

The process of motivation is a complex one, that has been studied and pondered over the ages. Throughout all of this study we have learned a number of valuable principles. These include:

- Human motivation is a process that evolves for each of us;
- No one item motivates all of us.
- What motivates us today may change tomorrow, based on competing forces that are internal and external to our experiences of life.

Let's Begin

Let's get back to looking at your present state of motivation. If you find that you are presently following your plan of change and that you are on the mark for moving forward, stick with your process. If you are struggling or maybe have stopped completely, now is the time to step back and look at your motivating factors.

A very important point to remember is that you have moved to this point in time. By deciding to read these words, you still are motivated to making a change in your health status. Let's use this opportunity to explore what is needed to continue to move forward with your process.

The key to our desire to change is based on our level of commitment to staying with the process. The spark for our commitment is a clear, compelling vision of what we want to create for ourselves.

The journey to health is not always a straight line. Health comes at different times and from different directions, and the key is to remain moving forward. Ask yourself these questions and ponder your answers:

- What have I learned about my motivational qualities, thus far into this process?

- Am I more internally motivated [I believe taking the necessary steps to being healthy is imperative] or am I more externally moti vated [the way I look is the most important result of being healthy].
- Do I need to team-up with someone or a group of individuals, to support each other with our changes?
- What were the barriers that I allowed to distract me from my stated commitment?
- Are they internal or external barriers?" What do I have to modify in my life to move beyond these barriers?
- Am I worth the push that it will take to recommit myself to living a healthy lifestyle?
- Knowing this information, am I ready to recommit myself to the necessary changes?
- What is my revised plan to allowing myself to move forward?
- What do I need to Start Doing? What do I need to Stop Doing… and what do I need to Continue Doing?

Step Seven

Remember, the key to commitment is a clear and compelling vision of what you want to create for your life. The future is not a place that is already set. It is a place that you create with your mind, then your heart, and then with your actions and behaviors.

Module Eight

Have you started to notice that your lifestyle is changing? Are the new habits you have been working on beginning to feel familiar?

Now can be a very important time in your efforts to make your changes permanent. Look at the goals you set at the start of this program. Have you met some of those goals already? Everyday struggles in life can be challenging, and the next technique you will be learning will help you through these struggles, helping you maintain your weight and lifestyle change.

Let's begin!

Stress, like food, is neither good nor bad; stress is just something that started when life began. We usually think that stress is bad for us, but actually, we couldn't maintain life without it. Hans Selye, who is identified as the father of stress management, discussed extensively the effects of stress and how the body responds. He identified two types of stress: eustress, and distress. Eustress is defined as positive stress and distress is defined as negative stress. Eustress promotes health while distress promotes illness.

Your body has only one way to respond to stress, whether it is eustress or distress. For example, your body will respond the same to both the birth of a child or the death of a loved one. Your body has a "fight or flight" response, meaning it is prepared to fight or run whenever it perceives that a stressor is harmful. The changes in the body that are produced by the "fight or flight" response include: increased pulse rate, sweating, shallow breathing, constricted blood flow, and changes in blood chemistry. Psychological changes include increased levels of anxiety and depression.

To help control these feelings, sometimes you find yourself turning to eating. Research has shown that eating carbohydrates, such as chips, candy, ice cream, chocolate, pie, cake, bread, or crackers, can actually help calm you down. This is a great relief when you can't seem to find relief otherwise. The consumption of the carbohydrates can help increase the amount of seratonin in the brain. Consuming proteins and fats doesn't have the same effect. Think about it - when was the last time you went looking for a piece of meat or a chicken leg when you were under stress?

Unfortunately, while being very effective, consuming carbohydrates under stress has a negative side effect…weight gain.

The following technique will give you something to use, instead of food, when you are feeling your stress level becoming negative.

The first step is to create a peaceful place in your mind for you to go to. This place can be a place that is familiar to you, or it can be something that you envision in your mind. The only rule of this place is that you are there by yourself. If there are people in the distance, they cannot be known to you. For example, if you see yourself on a beach, there may be people on a boardwalk behind you, but no one whom you know.

Some examples of this location could be floating on a raft in a quiet lake; sitting in a favorite chair, reading a book; walking through the woods on a crisp fall day; swinging on a swing in the park; sitting on a bench by a stream; or riding a horse through a field of grass.

Take a few minutes and think of where this place is for you. You may find, in the future, that you change it, but for now, simply pick a place.

Now, draw a picture of this special place, or describe this location as best you can. Take the time to write down everything about this location. This will be very important in the future. Use all of your senses to record this place: What do you see, taste, hear, feel and smell? If you are at the ocean, do you hear the seagulls, taste the salty air, smell the fish, see the waves and feel the sand under your feet? Take as much time as you need to make this location just as vivid as you can.

The next step is to begin to relax the body. Our bodies tense up when they are stressed, and sometimes we are not even aware of it. We are going to start at our toes and tighten and relax all the muscles of our bodies. It will be a simple exercise, but as with all exercises, it is important to obtain permission from your physician.

Find a chair, or a spot on the floor, where you can be comfortable. Ideally, you are not wearing confining clothing, and it is neither too hot nor too cold. Uncross your legs and arms, and take a few deep breaths. Relaxed breathing is very important to total relaxation. You can keep your eyes open or closed for this exercise.

Start with tightening all the muscles in your toes, and then tighten the muscles in your feet, in your calves, in your thighs, and finally your buttocks. Make them very tight, and hold them for the count of five. Then, starting with your buttocks, moving next to your thighs, your calves, your feet and finally your toes, slowly relax the muscles, feeling the warmth of the blood as the muscles begin to relax. Notice how warm your legs and feet feel. Feel the sensation of relaxation all through your legs - all the tension leaving your legs and, in its place, just a great feeling of warmth and relaxation.

Next, tighten the muscles in your back, your abdomen, your chest and your shoulders. Make them very tight, and hold them for the count of five. Then, starting with your back, moving next to your abdomen, your chest and your shoulders, slowly relax the muscles, feeling the warmth of the blood as the muscles begin to relax. Notice how warm your back, abdomen, chest and shoulders feel. Feel the sensation of relaxation all through your back, abdomen, chest and shoulders - all the tension leaving and, in its place, just a great feeling of warmth and relaxation.

Now, tighten the muscles in your neck and face. Make all the muscles very tight and hold them for the count of five. Then, starting with your neck and moving next to your face, slowly relax the muscles, feeling the warmth of the blood as the muscles begin to relax. Notice how warm your neck and face feel. Feel the sensation of relaxation all through your neck and face - all the tension leaving and, in its place, just a great feeling of warmth and relaxation.

Feel the warmth and relaxation all over your body. How does your body feel? Can you identify any spots that still hold tension? If you do, try slowly tightening that area and relaxing it again.

Now, while you are feeling relaxed, recall that place which you wrote about. See it in full detail. Use your senses and make the place come alive for you. Associate your feeling of relaxation with the picture you are now seeing. Try not to fall asleep. Feel relaxed.

Now, slowly open your eyes, and realize that you are still here, but now feeling much more relaxed, and in control.

You may want to record this script, either in your own voice, or someone else's voice which you find comfortable and relaxing. Practice this exercise three times a day, and, in a short period of time, you will start to notice that you only have to think of your picture and your body will start to relax.

Quick Relaxation Tips

- Get in a relaxed position.
- Take two deep cleaning breaths.
- Tense toes, legs, buttocks – hold – relax.
- Tense hands, arms, shoulders – hold – relax.

- Tense stomach, chest, pull shoulders back – hold – relax.
- Tense facial muscles – hold – relax.
- Visualize your favorite scene.
- Feel yourself relaxed and in control.
- Open your eyes – Go on with your day.

Step Eight

Eating is one way to manage stress, but unfortunately has the negative side effect of weight gain. When you find yourself eating, as a result of emotional stress, remove yourself to a quiet corner and use your relaxation technique to bring your emotions and eating back into control.

Module Nine

Review

You have reached the end of this road, but this is not a "dead-end." Just like a road map, there are more roads and turns to make as you continue on your journey to good health. As William Butler Yeats wrote, "The journey internally, is not only an important journey, it is the only journey." Your life is now, in the moment, don't wait for tomorrow to begin. Live now!

Let's Begin

Too often we wait. Wait for the right conditions, the right time, the right weight. Learning to accept who you are, at the point at which you are at in your life, can be a difficult task, but one that brings many rewards.

Learning to accept your body, at whatever weight it is, is a struggle that many people wrestle with all their lives. Each one of us inherited a set of genes from our parents that determined, for example, the color of our eyes, the color of our hair, how tall we will be, and what size shoe we will wear. We usually accept these features and realize that, even though we may have wished to have brown eyes instead of blue, there's not much we can do, and we move on with our lives. But when it comes to our weight, we get stuck in wishing it were different and NOT being able to move on with our lives. We tell ourselves that we will wait to do things until we have reached our weight goal, and, if we don't reach that goal or decide when we get there that the goal isn't good enough, we wait some more.

Mark Twain had a wonderful saying:

***"Twenty years from now you will be more disappointed by the things that you didn't do than by the ones you did do.
So throw off the bowlines.
Sail away from the safe harbor.
Catch the trade winds in your sails.
Explore. Dream. Discover."***

-Mark Twain

Life is so much more than the number on the scale. Take a moment and reflect on the following poem that was written by Mother Teresa.

Just Do It

People are often unreasonable, illogical, and self-centered;
Forgive them anyway.
If you are kind, people may accuse you of selfish, ulterior motives; Be kind anyway.
If you are successful, you will win some false friends and some true enemies; Succeed anyway.
If you are honest and frank, people may cheat you ; Be honest and frank anyway.
What you spend years building, someone could destroy overnight; Build anyway.
If you find serenity and happiness, they may be jealous; Be happy anyway.
The good you do today, people will often forget tomorrow; Do good anyway.
Give the world the best you have, and it may never be enough;
Give the world the best you've got anyway.
You see, in the final analysis, it is between you and God; It was never between you and them anyway.

There are some questions to consider, as you evaluate your body acceptance. We would like you to answer the questions, and, if you feel comfortable, share them with us:

- What definition do you use to define "beauty?"
- Where did you learn the definition?
- Would you apply the definition to someone you love?
- How do you fit into the definition?
- Do you have a different standard of beauty for yourself than for those you care about?
- Does your definition need to be modified? If so, in what ways?
- What do you need to do first, to become more accepting of your body?

These are important questions. We would like to hear from you regarding the first step you are planning to take to improve your body acceptance.

You have spent a lot of time working on modifying your lifestyle. You are to be congratulated!

You have adjusted your meal times, carved out time to be active, planned meals and are going grocery shopping. Go back again and review all the chapters.

Step Nine

Stay in touch, or move to the next level, and continue to learn and explore more healthy enhancing techniques.

Biographies

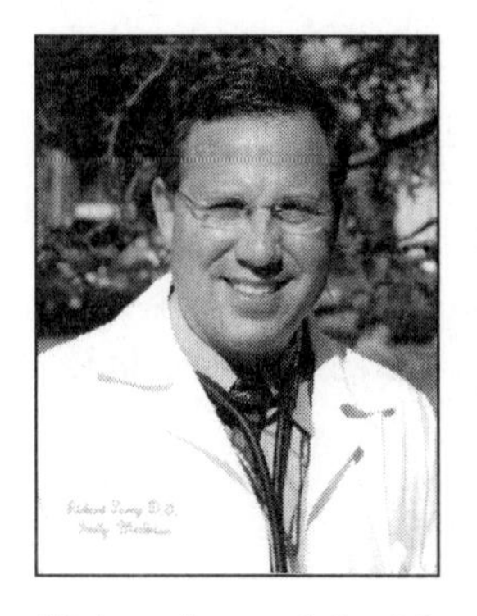

Dr. Richard Terry is a 1988 graduate of the New York College of Osteopathic Medicine in Old Westbury, New York. He completed a one year rotating internship at the Interfaith Medical Center in Brooklyn, New York and completed his residency in Family Practice at the University of Rochester/Highland Hospital in Rochester, New York.

Dr. Terry is a clinical associate professor of Family Medicine at SUNY Upstate Medical University and the New York College of Osteopathic Medicine. He is also the Director of Osteopathic Medical Education and Director of the Wilson Family Practice Residency program.

Dr. Terry has lectured both regionally and nationally on the subject of Obesity and also is the editor of the Obesity section in the Dyna Med - Dynamic Medical Information System. Dr. Terry is also a contributing author in the Essentials of Family Practice, edited by Robert E. Rakel, MD - 2004.

Dr. Terry is the Medical Director of Medical Nutrition Consulting.

Dr. Terry is an avid runner and has completed seven marathons. He resides in Apalachin, New York with his wife and four children.

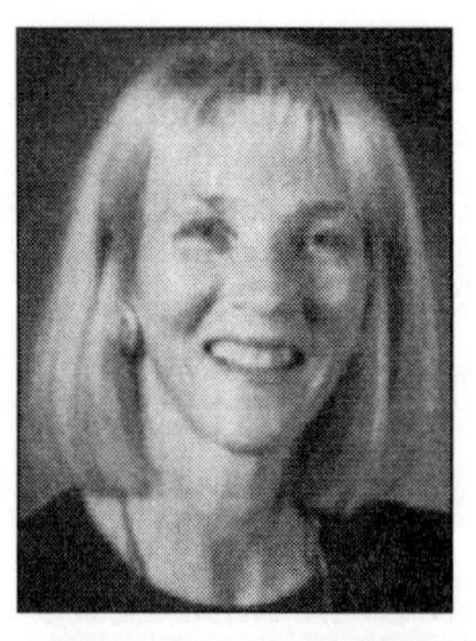

Helen Battisti, MS, RD, is the CNO of Medical Nutrition Consulting, a multi-disciplinary facility that specializes in nutrition intervention. She is an adjunct professor at the Marywood University Graduate School, Scranton, PA, and State University of New York - Broome Community College.

Mrs. Battisti's practice emphasizes preventative nutrition therapy that focuses on sports/performance, health enhancement, disease-prevention and control. Her dynamic style has made her a-much-sought-after presenter and lecturer. Helen is also anchor of a weekly Nutrition Segment on Fox 40 news, in Binghamton NY. She lives in upstate NY with her husband and three sons and is a marathon runner.

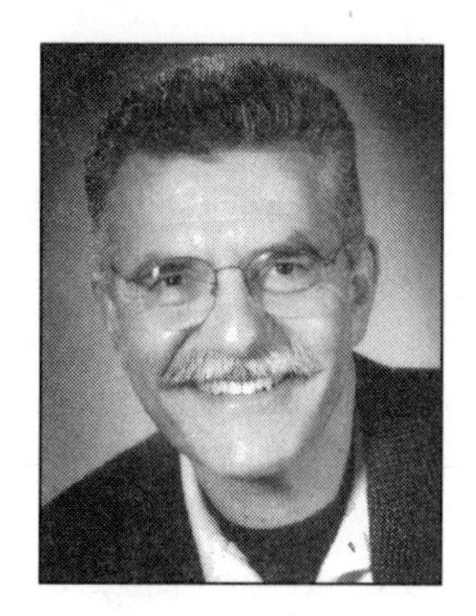

Francis L. Battisti, LCSW, BCD, is the CEO of Battisti Network, a multi-discipline consulting firm specializing in individual and organizational transformation and life enhancement. He is a Clinical Social Worker in private practice and Professor of Psychology and Human Services at the State University of New York - Broome Community College Campus where he was the recipient of the State University of New York Chancellor's Award for Excellence in Teaching.

Francis' impressive credentials as a seminar presenter and keynoter are highlighted by national and international appearances for Fortune 500 companies, small businesses, health organizations, educational institutions and national conventions. He offers participants a panoramic pathway to live with passion and spontaneity, as well as to trust their intuition. Francis is the author of a number of videos and audio-tapes and the forthcoming books, "Checchino: A Father and Son Journey Toward Dusk."

Francis lives in upstate New York with his wife and three sons. Francis is also a marathon runner.